The Business of American Healthcare

Why It Works and Who It Works For

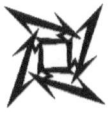

The Business of American Healthcare – Why It Works and Who It Works For
Copyright © 2024 by Angel Marqués
All rights reserved.

No part of this book may be reproduced, stored in a retrieval system, or transmitted in any form or by any means—electronic, mechanical, photocopying, recording, or otherwise—without prior written permission from the author, except in the case of brief quotations for book reviews or similar purposes permitted by copyright law.

This is a work of non-fiction. All content and interpretations herein are based on research and analysis by the author. Any resemblance to real persons, living or dead, is purely coincidental.

Published by Angel Marqués Sánchez
ISBN: **9798304031516**

Hello! I would greatly appreciate it if you could share your opinion by leaving a review on Amazon. Reviews not only help other readers discover the book, but they're also essential for supporting future projects.

If you have a few minutes, please visit the review page by scanning the QR code below.

The U.S. healthcare system stands as one of the great paradoxes of the modern world. Within its framework lies a duality that both awes and frustrates—cutting-edge advancements capable of saving lives are often inaccessible to those who need them most. For those fortunate enough to navigate its labyrinthine complexities with sufficient resources, the system provides unparalleled care. Yet, for millions, it represents a maze of unaffordable treatments, denied coverage, and relentless bureaucracy. It is a system that both inspires hope and breeds despair, and the tension between these realities defines its existence. The recent killing of UnitedHealthcare CEO Brian Thompson, though shocking in its details, has become a grim metaphor for the forces at play within this industry—a stark reminder of the stakes, the power struggles, and the human cost that permeate the business of care.

Thompson's death, while an extreme and singular event, underscores the fraught terrain of healthcare in America. It is a system driven not merely by the imperative to heal but also by the pursuit of profit, where corporate interests intersect with human vulnerability in ways that can be both transformative and destructive. The act of care, once a deeply personal exchange between doctor and patient, now unfolds against the backdrop of financial calculations, legal constraints, and political maneuvering. In this context, Thompson's story becomes more than just a tragedy—it becomes a lens through which we might begin to unravel the complex forces that shape this system and dictate for whom it truly works.

The paradox of American healthcare is not accidental, nor is it entirely unique. It is the product of a system deeply intertwined with the country's values, its history, and its political ideologies. Built on principles of innovation and individualism, it thrives in areas where ingenuity and competition are paramount. But these same forces also create fissures, exposing fault lines that manifest as inequality, inefficiency, and moral ambiguity. The very structures that allow some to access life-saving treatments consign others to neglect, offering a sobering reflection of the broader economic and social hierarchies that define American life.

To examine this system is to confront uncomfortable truths about the intersection of morality, economics, and power. For decades, political ideologies have clashed over the role of government in healthcare, with proponents of free-market solutions emphasizing efficiency and innovation while critics point to the human toll of leaving care to the whims of market forces. Yet, even as the debate rages on, the system continues to operate with remarkable consistency—offering much to those who can afford it while demanding impossible compromises from those who cannot. It is not a system that has failed, but one that functions exactly as designed.

Fundamentally, the U.S. healthcare system is a mirror, reflecting the values and priorities of the society that sustains it. This book begins with a simple yet profound question: If this system represents what America values most, what does that say about the nation and its future? The answer lies not in seeking simplistic solutions or vilifying its architects, but in understanding the deeper forces at work—the historical, economic, and political currents that have shaped this paradoxical institution. As we delve into its evolution, its beneficiaries, and its casualties, we are left to wrestle with the uncomfortable reality that, for all its flaws, this system remains profoundly American.

THE PARADOX OF CARE 7

PART 1: THE BIRTH OF A HEALTHCARE INDUSTRY 17

Chapter 1: Early Roots - Healthcare Before It Was a Business 18
Chapter 2: Medicare, Medicaid, and the Expansion of State Involvement ... 25
Chapter 3: The Free Market Takes Over 42

PART 2: A SYSTEM OF WINNERS AND LOSERS 67

Chapter 4: The Business of Medicine - Who Profits, Who Pays 68
Chapter 5: The Disparities of Care 83
Chapter 6: The Human Cost of Profit-Driven Care 102

PART 3: POLITICS, POLICY, AND POWER 115

Chapter 7: Healthcare as a Political Battlefield 116
Chapter 8: The Lobbyists' Playground 141
Chapter 9: Reform or Rhetoric? The Cycles of Healthcare Debate 164

PART 4: THE FUTURE OF HEALTHCARE IN AMERICA 181

Chapter 10: The Role of Technology - A Cure or a Band-Aid? 182
Chapter 11: Privatization vs. Universal Care - What's Next? 194
Chapter 12: The Global Lens - Lessons from Other Countries 206
Chapter 13: Healthcare That Works - Without Breaking the System 226
Chapter 14: Reimagining Responsibility - Government, Corporations, and the Individual 243
Chapter 15: The Cost of Inaction 254

A HEALTHCARE SYSTEM AMERICA DESERVES 268

DISCOVER MORE 276

The Paradox of Care

The United States healthcare system embodies a profound paradox: it is simultaneously one of the most innovative and inequitable systems in the world. It produces groundbreaking advancements that push the boundaries of medical science, offering treatments that can extend life, alleviate suffering, and cure diseases that were once fatal. Yet these achievements coexist with staggering levels of exclusion, where access to this innovation is rationed by socioeconomic status, geography, and insurance coverage. The system saves lives in spectacular ways, but only for those who can afford its price, leaving millions in the shadow of its success. This contradiction is not merely a flaw in its design but a feature embedded in its foundation—a reflection of the ideological and economic forces that have shaped its trajectory.

On one hand, the U.S. has become a global leader in medical technology, pharmaceutical development, and clinical research. Its hospitals are home to world-renowned specialists, and its biotech industry drives a significant portion of global innovation. But these accomplishments are not universally shared. For the uninsured, the underinsured, or those burdened by exorbitant medical debt, these advancements remain distant and unattainable. The care that is meant to heal is distributed through a filter of cost-effectiveness and profit margins, where the ability to pay determines the quality and availability of treatment.

This paradox is most visible in the stories of those left behind by the system. Families forced into bankruptcy due to medical expenses, patients denied life-saving treatments because of policy loopholes, and rural communities unable to sustain even a single hospital—all of these point to the stark inequities embedded in a system that is celebrated for its excellence. These stories are not exceptions but symptoms of a broader structural imbalance. The healthcare system works, but it works selectively—exceptionally well for some, devastatingly poorly for others.

What makes this paradox particularly striking is the ideological justification that sustains it. The U.S. healthcare system is rooted in a philosophy that prioritizes individual choice, competition, and innovation, often at the expense of collective welfare. Proponents argue that market-driven solutions foster efficiency and encourage innovation, and indeed, the system delivers extraordinary results in areas where profit incentives align with medical progress. Yet, this same market logic creates blind spots, ignoring those whose needs cannot be neatly monetized or whose care would not yield a profitable return. The system's successes are inseparable from its failures, and its greatest strengths are intertwined with its deepest flaws.

Critics often label the U.S. healthcare system as "broken," but this characterization misses the deeper truth: the system is not broken—it is performing exactly as designed. It functions within the framework of capitalism, where the allocation of resources is dictated by market dynamics rather than universal need. The result is a system that excels in areas where wealth and access converge while systematically marginalizing those who fall outside these parameters. This is not an accident but a reflection of the nation's broader values and priorities, where the ideals of innovation and individualism are often placed above equity and accessibility.

To understand the paradox of care in America is to grapple with the uncomfortable reality that the system's inequities are not aberrations but integral to its operation. It is a system that inspires admiration and outrage in equal measure, embodying both the heights of human achievement and the depths of societal disparity. This tension lies at the heart of the U.S. healthcare debate, raising fundamental questions about who the system serves, who it excludes, and what it says about the nation as a whole. In this paradox, we find not only the story of American healthcare but also a reflection of the larger societal contradictions that define the country itself.

THE POLITICAL AND CORPORATE FORCES

The U.S. healthcare system is a battleground where political ideologies and corporate interests converge, shaping not only the way care is delivered but also the lives of millions who depend on it. At its core, the system is both a product of and a participant in the nation's larger political and economic dynamics. Its evolution is marked by intense lobbying, policy decisions swayed by financial power, and a deep entanglement between government and private enterprise. These forces do not merely influence the system—they define its very structure, ensuring that healthcare in America remains an arena where profit and policy are inseparable.

From the earliest days of employer-sponsored insurance to the passage of the Affordable Care Act, the healthcare system has been shaped by ideological battles over the role of government versus the free market. Conservatives have long championed a minimal government approach, advocating for market-driven solutions that emphasize competition and personal responsibility. Liberals, by contrast, have pushed for broader public programs and regulatory oversight to address inequities and expand access to care. Yet, despite their stark differences, both sides have ultimately allowed corporate interests to dominate the system, often framing their policies in ways that benefit powerful industry stakeholders while marginalizing the needs of ordinary citizens.

Nowhere is this dynamic more evident than in the influence of the pharmaceutical and insurance industries, which wield immense power over the legislative and regulatory process. With billions of dollars spent annually on lobbying and political campaigns, these industries have successfully shaped policies that protect their profit margins, often at the expense of patient care. From skyrocketing drug prices to opaque insurance practices that leave consumers baffled and vulnerable, corporate priorities have become deeply embedded in the fabric of the system. It is a system designed to thrive in profitability, even as it falters in its promise of universal care.

The killing of UnitedHealthcare CEO Brian Thompson serves as a harrowing illustration of the tensions that arise in such a deeply monetized environment. While Thompson's death is not representative of the daily operations of the industry, it highlights the profound disconnect between the corporate leadership that drives the healthcare system and the public it is meant to serve. CEOs like Thompson navigate a precarious balancing act: driving shareholder value while grappling with public outrage over perceived greed and systemic inequities. This dual role, as both the face of innovation and the target of resentment, underscores the fraught relationship between healthcare as a business and healthcare as a human right.

The political landscape surrounding healthcare further complicates this dynamic. Policy decisions, often driven by short-term electoral considerations, frequently leave systemic issues unaddressed. Debates over Medicare expansion, drug price negotiations, and health equity are reduced to partisan soundbites, while long-term reform remains elusive. Politicians on both sides of the aisle are incentivized to preserve the status quo, either out of ideological commitment to free-market principles or reliance on campaign contributions from healthcare corporations. The result is a system in perpetual stasis, where incremental changes are celebrated as monumental victories, even as millions continue to fall through the cracks.

Despite these challenges, political and corporate forces are not merely obstacles—they are also opportunities. The same entities that profit from the system's inequities have the power to drive change, provided there is sufficient pressure from consumers, advocates, and policymakers. The question is whether the system's architects are willing to embrace a model that prioritizes health outcomes over revenue. History suggests that this will not happen without significant public and political will, yet the growing outcry over healthcare costs and access suggests that change may be inevitable, even if incremental.

The U.S. healthcare system is a reflection of the broader societal relationship between power, profit, and policy. It is a system that operates within the constraints of capitalism, where political ideologies and corporate interests are not separate from care but are intrinsic to its operation. To examine these forces is to uncover the underlying mechanisms that dictate who receives care, who profits from its provision, and what the future of American healthcare might hold. In this exploration, we confront the uncomfortable reality that the system's failures are not anomalies but the natural outcome of a structure that prioritizes economic and political power over human need.

The Capitalist Argument

The U.S. healthcare system is often held up as a quintessential example of capitalism at work—both its achievements and its shortcomings. Proponents of the capitalist argument contend that competition and market forces drive innovation, efficiency, and choice, positioning the United States as a global leader in medical advancements. Yet, this same market logic has created a system where access to care often depends more on financial resources than on medical necessity. The result is a paradoxical landscape where the highest quality care in the world exists alongside some of the deepest inequities.

At the heart of the capitalist defense is the notion that markets, when left to function freely, incentivize innovation and optimize resource allocation. The U.S. healthcare system undeniably excels in certain areas: it boasts world-class research institutions, cutting-edge medical technology, and pharmaceutical breakthroughs that have revolutionized treatment for diseases once considered fatal. Advocates argue that this progress is a direct result of competition, where private companies and research entities strive for excellence to gain market share and deliver shareholder returns. In this view, the privatized model is not a flaw but a feature—a necessary mechanism for maintaining the dynamism that drives medical progress.

However, the capitalist argument also hinges on the belief that consumer choice ensures accountability. Patients, as consumers, are theoretically empowered to select from a range of providers, insurance plans, and treatments, forcing companies to compete on cost and quality. Yet, in practice, this ideal rarely materializes. Healthcare consumers often face opaque pricing structures, limited provider networks, and a lack of transparency that undermines informed decision-making. The commodification of care creates an environment where the "customer" is frequently at a disadvantage, navigating a system designed more for corporate gain than for patient empowerment.

Critics of the capitalist model point to the inherent tension between profit motives and the ethical imperatives of care. In a market-driven system, the primary goal of stakeholders—insurance companies, hospital systems, pharmaceutical corporations—is to maximize profits. This often leads to cost-cutting measures, denial of coverage, and exorbitant pricing practices that prioritize shareholder value over patient outcomes. The consequences are stark: medical bankruptcy remains a uniquely American phenomenon, and millions of uninsured and underinsured individuals are excluded from receiving adequate care. For many, the capitalist argument rings hollow when the promise of innovation comes at the cost of widespread inaccessibility.

Nevertheless, defenders of the capitalist framework counter that the system's inequities are not inherent to capitalism itself but rather the result of insufficient competition and overregulation. They argue that government intervention, through programs like Medicare and Medicaid or regulations imposed by the Affordable Care Act, distorts market dynamics and entrenches inefficiencies. From this perspective, the solution is not less capitalism but more: deregulation, price transparency, and increased competition among providers and insurers would, they claim, lead to a more equitable and efficient system. This view posits that the free market can and should be the ultimate arbiter of value in healthcare, capable of delivering both innovation and accessibility when properly incentivized.

The capitalist argument also draws strength from its alignment with American cultural values, particularly individualism and self-reliance. It reinforces the belief that individuals should bear responsibility for their health and that access to care is, at least in part, a function of personal effort and economic contribution. This ethos underpins employer-sponsored insurance models and the emphasis on health savings accounts, which place greater financial responsibility—and risk—on individuals. For many, the capitalist model is not only an economic framework but a moral one, reflecting a deeply ingrained belief in meritocracy and personal accountability.

Yet, this alignment with cultural values also exposes the system's moral contradictions. While the capitalist model rewards innovation and personal agency, it often fails to account for structural inequalities that leave large segments of the population without adequate care. In a system driven by profit, the most vulnerable—those with chronic illnesses, low incomes, or unstable employment—are systematically disadvantaged. The question, then, is whether a healthcare system rooted in capitalist principles can reconcile its pursuit of profit with the moral obligation to provide care for all.

The capitalist argument for healthcare is compelling in its emphasis on innovation, efficiency, and choice. It captures the aspirational elements of the American ethos, presenting the market as both a driver of progress and a mechanism for accountability. However, it also lays bare the ethical dilemmas and systemic failures that arise when care is commodified. Whether capitalism is the solution or the problem depends on one's perspective, but what is clear is that the U.S. healthcare system embodies the tensions inherent in applying market principles to a domain as fundamentally human as health. This chapter seeks to unravel these tensions, exploring how capitalism shapes the system's successes and shortcomings and what this means for its future.

The Origins of a Fragmented System

The roots of the U.S. healthcare system's current state lie not in a singular, deliberate design but in a patchwork of policies, cultural values, and historical contingencies that have evolved over centuries. To understand why the system functions as it does today, it is essential to trace its origins, examining the economic, political, and societal forces that laid the groundwork for a healthcare model as fragmented as it is formidable.

Unlike many other developed nations, where centralized healthcare systems emerged as deliberate responses to social needs, the American system grew out of a laissez-faire ethos that prized individual autonomy and minimal government intervention. In the 19th and early 20th centuries, healthcare was largely a private affair, with medical care provided by individual practitioners, community hospitals, and charitable organizations. There was no unified structure, no comprehensive safety net—only a disparate array of services that varied widely in quality and accessibility, largely influenced by geography, race, and class.

The rise of employer-sponsored health insurance during World War II marked a pivotal turning point, embedding healthcare within the fabric of the labor market. Faced with wage freezes during the war, employers began offering health benefits as a way to attract and retain workers, setting the stage for the dominance of private insurance. What began as a pragmatic solution to a wartime problem became the bedrock of the American healthcare system, tying access to care to employment and creating a profound divide between those who had insurance and those who did not.

As the system grew, so too did its complexity. The introduction of Medicare and Medicaid in the 1960s was a landmark moment, addressing the needs of the elderly, disabled, and low-income populations left behind by the employer-based model. These programs were transformative, yet they also reinforced the system's duality, carving out separate paths for public and private care rather than creating a unified approach. This division entrenched a system where healthcare access depended as much on political negotiation and economic status as on medical need.

Throughout the late 20th century, the commercialization of healthcare accelerated, further splintering the system. Hospitals merged into sprawling health systems, pharmaceutical companies expanded their influence, and insurers became powerful gatekeepers of care. The industry's increasing corporatization prioritized efficiency and profitability, often at the expense of equitable access. Meanwhile, attempts at reform—most notably the Affordable Care Act—have sought to bridge gaps without fundamentally restructuring the system, layering new policies atop an already fractured foundation.

This fragmented history has left the U.S. healthcare system at once innovative and inequitable, efficient in some respects and woefully inefficient in others. It is a system where extraordinary medical breakthroughs coexist with inaccessibility and systemic disparities, where care is both celebrated for its excellence and criticized for its exclusivity. These contradictions are not incidental but foundational, the result of decades of piecemeal decisions that prioritized market dynamics, political expediency, and cultural individualism over universal access.

Understanding this history is crucial for setting the stage. It allows us to see the system not as an immutable monolith but as a living entity, shaped by the forces of its time and open to transformation. The fragmented foundation of American healthcare explains not only its present complexities but also its vulnerabilities, offering insight into how the system might evolve—or unravel—in the years ahead. By exploring these origins, we begin to grasp the full scope of what is at stake in the ongoing struggle to reconcile the promise of care with the reality of its delivery.

Part 1: The Birth of a Healthcare Industry

Chapter 1: Early Roots – Healthcare Before It Was a Business

In early America, healthcare was a communal endeavor, rooted in the moral values and social fabric of the time. It was not viewed as a commodity to be bought and sold, but as a shared responsibility, often tied to religious and philanthropic efforts. Churches, charitable organizations, and local communities played a central role in providing care to the sick and needy. Hospitals, when they existed, were rudimentary and largely served as shelters for the destitute or as places for those suffering from infectious diseases. Institutions like Pennsylvania Hospital, founded in 1751 with the help of Benjamin Franklin, exemplified this early model of charitable care. These hospitals relied heavily on donations, public subscriptions, and volunteer support, operating as extensions of the community's moral and ethical commitment to care for its members.

The ethos of healthcare as a moral duty was deeply embedded in the religious underpinnings of American society. Judeo-Christian values emphasized charity and service to others, and caring for the sick was seen as a natural extension of these beliefs. Physicians, when available, often provided services either without charge or at minimal cost, motivated by a sense of duty rather than financial gain. Communities took collective responsibility for their vulnerable members, pooling resources to ensure that no one was entirely abandoned in times of illness. However, this system had its limits. Access to care was uneven, and many marginalized groups, including enslaved individuals, Indigenous populations, and the poorest of the poor, were excluded from even these basic forms of assistance. Healthcare, while altruistic in its intentions, was constrained by the lack of medical knowledge and the limited resources available in these early years.

As the nineteenth century unfolded, the landscape of healthcare began to change. The professionalization of medicine marked a significant shift in how care was delivered. Organizations like the American Medical Association, established in 1847, sought to standardize medical education and practice, elevating the status of physicians and formalizing their role within society. This professionalization also introduced market dynamics into the healthcare system. Physicians, who had once worked within the communal and charitable framework, began to charge fees for their services, and the relationship between doctor and patient became more transactional. With this shift came a growing disparity in access to care. Those who could afford private practitioners received better treatment, while others were left to rely on overburdened charitable institutions or self-care.

The limitations of charitable care became more apparent as the U.S. grew into an industrialized nation. Urbanization and population growth stretched the capacity of local hospitals and community-based models. At the same time, advances in medical science created new opportunities for treatment but also increased the costs of providing care. This period laid the groundwork for the commodification of healthcare, as the need for sustainable funding models began to outweigh the altruistic ideals of earlier years.

After World War II, the transformation of healthcare accelerated with the rise of employer-provided insurance. During the war, federal wage controls prevented companies from increasing salaries, leading many employers to offer health benefits as a form of indirect compensation. The federal government encouraged this practice by exempting these benefits from taxation, effectively embedding employer-sponsored insurance into the American healthcare system. This shift marked a decisive break from the communal ethos of earlier eras. Healthcare was no longer a moral responsibility shared by society but a benefit tied to one's employment, further stratifying access based on socioeconomic status.

The rise of employer-sponsored insurance created a dual system: one for those who worked in industries offering comprehensive benefits and another for those left uninsured or underinsured. For many, this shift represented progress, as it expanded access to medical care and facilitated advancements in treatments and technologies. But it also deepened inequities, creating a system in which access to healthcare became increasingly dependent on one's job, income, and employer. This model, while innovative, entrenched a profit-driven approach to healthcare delivery, paving the way for the privatized and fragmented system that would define the U.S. healthcare landscape in the decades to come.

The evolution from charitable care to employer-provided insurance reflects broader shifts in American society, including the rise of capitalism and the prioritization of individualism over collective welfare. It underscores how economic and political forces shaped the foundation of modern healthcare, transforming it from a communal obligation into an industry defined by profit and access disparities. While the early system was far from perfect, its moral and communal underpinnings offer a stark contrast to the commercialized reality that would follow.

The Rise of Private Practitioners

The rise of private practitioners in the United States marked a pivotal moment in the evolution of healthcare, reshaping the relationship between providers and patients and laying the groundwork for the commodification of care. In the early 19th century, medicine in America began to shift from a community-centered practice rooted in charity and moral obligation to a professionalized field driven by individual practitioners seeking to establish their expertise and livelihoods. This transformation was catalyzed by a confluence of social, economic, and scientific changes that redefined the role of the physician and the nature of medical practice.

The professionalization of medicine emerged as a direct response to the disorganized and inconsistent state of healthcare during the early years of the republic. At the time, anyone could claim to be a doctor, and medical practice was largely unregulated. Quackery and unproven remedies were rampant, eroding public trust in medical practitioners. To address this, the American Medical Association (AMA) was founded in 1847 with the goal of standardizing medical education and raising the standards of medical practice. The AMA played a critical role in establishing licensure requirements and advocating for the creation of medical schools, effectively narrowing the field to trained and certified physicians. By formalizing the profession, medicine gained legitimacy and authority, elevating the status of physicians in American society.

As physicians professionalized, their services became more individualized and transactional. Private practitioners set up offices and began charging fees for their expertise, a departure from the charitable or communal models that had previously defined care. This shift represented a significant departure from the earlier ethos of healthcare as a shared responsibility. For many, the ability to pay for medical services became the determining factor in access to quality care. Wealthier patients could afford regular consultations, while poorer individuals relied on sporadic charity care or self-treatment. The introduction of a fee-for-service model not only changed the economics of healthcare but also altered the physician-patient dynamic, positioning the doctor as both a caregiver and a businessperson.

The rise of private practitioners also coincided with broader economic and social changes in the United States. Urbanization and industrialization created a growing middle class with the financial means to pay for medical services. This newfound wealth, combined with the professionalization of medicine, fostered a demand for more specialized and advanced care. Physicians capitalized on these opportunities, often focusing their practices in urban areas where they could attract wealthier clients. Rural communities, by contrast, were left underserved, as the economic incentives for private practice did not align with the needs of sparsely populated areas. This urban-rural divide further highlighted the disparities in access to care that began to emerge during this period.

Scientific advancements also played a critical role in the rise of private practitioners. The late 19th and early 20th centuries saw significant breakthroughs in medical knowledge, including the development of germ theory, the introduction of anesthesia, and the emergence of surgical techniques that were safer and more effective. These advancements increased the demand for trained physicians and further elevated their status in society. However, they also increased the cost of medical care, as doctors needed to invest in education, training, and equipment to stay current with the latest practices. These costs were inevitably passed on to patients, deepening the financial barriers to accessing care.

Despite the progress brought by professionalization, the rise of private practitioners highlighted the inherent tensions between healthcare as a public good and healthcare as a private enterprise. The transition to a fee-based system created clear winners and losers. Those who could afford to pay for private services benefited from improved care and the latest medical advancements, while those without financial means were left behind. This period also laid the foundation for the dominance of market dynamics in healthcare, as physicians and medical institutions increasingly prioritized financial sustainability over equitable access.

By the early 20th century, the private practice model had become the cornerstone of American healthcare. The physician was no longer a community servant but an independent entrepreneur, navigating the complexities of both medicine and commerce. This transformation reflected broader societal shifts toward individualism and capitalism, embedding these values within the very fabric of the healthcare system. While the professionalization of medicine undoubtedly improved the quality and consistency of care, it also introduced new challenges, particularly in ensuring that care was accessible to all, regardless of socioeconomic status.

The rise of private practitioners marked a critical juncture in the history of American healthcare, setting the stage for the commodification of medicine and the inequities that continue to define the system. It was a period of profound change, characterized by advancements in science and professional standards, but also by the growing influence of market forces. As private practitioners solidified their role as key players in the healthcare landscape, they laid the groundwork for the profit-driven model that would come to dominate the 20th century, shaping the trajectory of American healthcare for decades to come.

Employer-Provided Insurance Post-WWII

The advent of employer-provided health insurance in the United States after World War II was a transformative development that reshaped the healthcare landscape and solidified the link between employment and access to medical care. This shift did not occur in isolation but was the result of a series of historical, economic, and political factors that converged during the mid-20th century, forever altering the way healthcare was financed and delivered in America.

During World War II, the federal government implemented wage controls to curb inflation in a booming wartime economy. These controls prevented employers from offering higher salaries to attract workers, creating significant challenges for industries that needed to compete for labor in an era of full employment. To circumvent these restrictions, employers began to offer fringe benefits, including health insurance, as an alternative form of compensation. This practice was further incentivized in 1943 when the Internal Revenue Service ruled that employer contributions to health insurance premiums were not taxable as income. This decision created a powerful financial incentive for employers to provide health benefits, as it allowed them to offer attractive compensation packages without incurring additional tax liabilities.

By the end of the war, employer-sponsored health insurance had become firmly embedded in the American workplace. The expansion of this model was accelerated by labor unions, which began to negotiate health benefits as a key component of collective bargaining agreements. Unions saw health insurance as a critical means of improving workers' quality of life, and their advocacy helped to spread the practice across a broad range of industries. For employers, offering health benefits became a way to attract and retain talent in an increasingly competitive labor market, especially as the post-war economy transitioned to peacetime production.

The federal government further cemented this system through legislative actions in the 1950s. The codification of the tax exemption for employer sponsored health benefits in the Internal Revenue Code made these benefits even more advantageous for both employers and employees. This policy effectively subsidized private health insurance through forgone tax revenue, incentivizing its growth and entrenching it as the dominant method of healthcare financing in the United States.

The rise of employer-provided insurance also coincided with broader societal changes in post-war America. The rapid growth of the middle class, fueled by economic prosperity and suburbanization, created a population that was increasingly willing and able to pay for health services. Advances in medical technology and the expansion of hospital infrastructure, supported by programs like the Hill-Burton Act of 1946, further enhanced the value of health insurance, as it provided access to an ever-expanding array of treatments and procedures. The symbiosis between employer-sponsored insurance and the medical industry created a self-reinforcing cycle, driving both the demand for healthcare and its costs.

While employer-provided insurance brought significant benefits, such as expanded access to healthcare for millions of Americans, it also introduced structural inequities into the system. The reliance on employment as the primary gateway to health coverage meant that those without stable jobs—such as the unemployed, part-time workers, and those in the informal economy—were excluded from the system. These gaps disproportionately affected marginalized groups, including women, minorities, and low-income individuals, exacerbating existing disparities in access to care.

Moreover, the system's design tied healthcare coverage to one's job, creating a precarious situation for workers who lost their employment. The lack of portability in health insurance meant that a job loss often resulted in the loss of health coverage, leaving individuals vulnerable during periods of economic instability. This inherent instability became particularly evident during economic downturns, when unemployment spikes left millions without access to medical care.

The employer-provided insurance model also contributed to the fragmentation of the U.S. healthcare system. Unlike universal systems in other countries, which pool resources to provide coverage for all citizens, the American model created a patchwork of coverage that varied widely depending on one's employer, occupation, and geographic location. This fragmentation not only limited access for certain populations but also increased administrative complexity and costs, as insurers, employers, and providers navigated a maze of contracts, networks, and reimbursement mechanisms.

Despite its shortcomings, employer-provided insurance became deeply ingrained in American society, in part because it aligned with the nation's cultural and political values. The system's reliance on private markets and its emphasis on individual employment echoed broader capitalist ideals, reinforcing the notion that healthcare was a benefit earned through work rather than a universal right. Political efforts to expand coverage through alternative models, such as national health insurance, faced resistance from entrenched interests, including the insurance and healthcare industries, which benefited from the status quo.

By the mid-20th century, employer-provided insurance had become a defining feature of the American healthcare system, shaping its trajectory in profound ways. While it expanded access to care for millions, it also institutionalized inequities and inefficiencies that persist to this day. The model's reliance on employment as the foundation for health coverage created a system that was both innovative and inherently exclusionary, reflecting the broader tensions between capitalism, individualism, and collective welfare that continue to define the U.S. approach to healthcare.

CHAPTER 2: MEDICARE, MEDICAID, AND THE EXPANSION OF STATE INVOLVEMENT

The story of government involvement in healthcare begins with a paradox. On one hand, Medicare and Medicaid are hailed as two of the most significant achievements in modern American history, programs that symbolize compassion and equity by addressing the needs of the elderly, the poor, and the disabled. On the other hand, they are perennial sources of contention, fiercely debated for their costs, their perceived inefficiencies, and the ideological questions they raise about the role of government in a free-market society. The creation of these programs in the mid-20th century was a turning point, marking the federal government's most ambitious attempt to guarantee access to healthcare for its most vulnerable citizens. But this bold move came at a cost, reshaping not only how care is delivered and paid for but also how Americans view the very concept of healthcare.

In the years leading up to their enactment, the landscape of American healthcare was starkly different. Healthcare access was largely dependent on personal wealth or the benevolence of community-driven organizations. Hospitals operated on charity, and those who could afford private care often did so out of pocket. However, the economic growth following World War II and the rising costs of medical innovation began to leave increasing numbers of Americans behind. The elderly, particularly, faced a unique plight. As they retired and their incomes dwindled, so too did their ability to secure insurance or pay for rising healthcare expenses. These growing inequities called for intervention, and by the 1960s, the political winds were shifting toward reform. The Johnson administration, building on the New Deal ethos of its predecessors, sought to weave a safety net that would ensure healthcare as a basic right for these underserved groups. But the road to Medicare and Medicaid was anything but smooth.

The introduction of these programs was a flashpoint in the ongoing ideological struggle over the government's role in American life. Medicare, designed to provide health coverage for individuals over 65, was fiercely opposed by conservatives and industry stakeholders who decried it as a step toward socialism. Medicaid, which extended coverage to the poor through a federal-state partnership, faced its own set of challenges. While proponents celebrated these initiatives as victories for social justice, critics raised alarms about government overreach and fiscal sustainability. The debates surrounding their implementation foreshadowed many of the same arguments that continue to dominate healthcare reform today. From accusations of inefficiency to fears of entitlement culture, the rhetoric has endured, reflecting deep-seated tensions in the American psyche about individualism, responsibility, and the role of the state.

What Medicare and Medicaid accomplished was groundbreaking. For the first time, millions of Americans gained access to healthcare they would have otherwise been denied. Hospitals were integrated under the stipulation that they comply with civil rights legislation to receive federal funding, marking a significant step toward racial equality in healthcare. Physicians, once skeptical of government intervention, found themselves adjusting to the realities of reimbursement rates and standardized billing practices. Meanwhile, patients experienced the relief of knowing that age or poverty would no longer bar them from receiving care. But these programs were not without their flaws. The very structure of Medicaid, for instance, created disparities between states, where decisions on eligibility and benefits often mirrored local political climates. Medicare, though broadly successful, introduced complexities in cost management that would later become defining challenges for the system.

The legacy of these programs is both profound and complicated. They shifted public expectations of what healthcare should be, embedding the idea that the government has a moral obligation to protect its citizens from the catastrophic costs of illness. Yet, they also exposed the limits of such interventions, as rising costs, inefficiencies, and gaps in coverage continued to plague the system. These issues were not unforeseen; they were born out of compromises made during their inception, compromises that prioritized feasibility over perfection. As we delve deeper into the creation, impact, and enduring challenges of Medicare and Medicaid, it becomes clear that these programs are more than just policies. They are mirrors reflecting the values, contradictions, and aspirations of the society that birthed them.

The Birth of Medicare and Medicaid: A Historical Perspective

The origins of Medicare and Medicaid are steeped in the social and political upheavals of mid-20th century America, a time when the nation was grappling with the dual forces of progress and inequality. The post-World War II era ushered in unprecedented economic growth, technological advancements, and a burgeoning middle class. Yet, beneath this prosperity lay a glaring disparity: millions of Americans, particularly the elderly and the poor, were being excluded from the benefits of modern healthcare. Rising medical costs and the increasing specialization of care made healthcare less accessible to those without stable incomes or employer-provided insurance. This gap revealed the limits of market-driven solutions and set the stage for federal intervention.

The push for government-led healthcare reform was not a new phenomenon. Efforts to establish national health insurance had been debated since the

Progressive Era, with figures like Theodore Roosevelt and later Franklin D. Roosevelt championing the idea. However, these initiatives consistently faced resistance, primarily from powerful interest groups like the American Medical Association (AMA), which warned that such policies would lead to a loss of professional autonomy and the dreaded specter of "socialized medicine." By the 1960s, however, the climate had shifted. President Lyndon B. Johnson's Great Society agenda sought to address systemic inequities, from poverty to racial injustice, and healthcare reform became a cornerstone of this vision.

Medicare and Medicaid emerged from a contentious legislative process, one marked by compromise and political maneuvering. Medicare was conceived as a social insurance program modeled after Social Security, providing universal hospital and medical coverage for Americans over the age of 65. Its design reflected a careful balancing act: it offered broad benefits while ensuring that the program would be funded through payroll taxes, avoiding the perception of a direct welfare scheme. Medicaid, in contrast, was structured as a means-tested program, targeting low-income individuals and families. Unlike Medicare, it relied on a federal-state partnership, with states retaining significant control over eligibility and benefit design. This distinction would have profound implications for the long-term evolution of both programs.

The passage of the Social Security Amendments of 1965, which established Medicare and Medicaid, represented a legislative triumph but also highlighted the deep divisions in American society. The programs faced fierce opposition from conservative lawmakers and industry stakeholders, who argued that they infringed upon free-market principles and individual freedoms. At the same time, they were championed by civil rights activists, labor unions, and progressive policymakers, who viewed them as essential tools for achieving social justice. Johnson's administration leveraged public support, framing the programs as moral imperatives that aligned with the nation's democratic values. The result was a rare moment of bipartisan agreement, albeit one achieved through significant concessions to appease skeptics.

The implementation of Medicare and Medicaid was transformative. Medicare brought relief to millions of elderly Americans who had previously faced financial ruin or inadequate care due to medical expenses. It standardized hospital practices, increased access to advanced treatments, and incentivized the desegregation of healthcare facilities under Title VI of the Civil Rights Act. Medicaid, while more fragmented in its reach, provided a critical safety net for low-income populations, particularly children, pregnant women, and individuals with disabilities. Together, these programs reshaped the healthcare landscape, embedding the principle that certain populations have a right to medical care, regardless of their economic circumstances.

However, the programs also sowed the seeds of future challenges. The reliance on state administration for Medicaid created a patchwork of coverage, with stark disparities in access and quality depending on geography. Medicare's fee-for-service model encouraged rapid growth in healthcare spending, as providers were reimbursed for the volume rather than the value of services. These unintended consequences reflected the compromises inherent in their design, compromises that prioritized immediate feasibility over long-term sustainability. Nonetheless, the birth of Medicare and Medicaid marked a watershed moment in American history, setting a precedent for government intervention in a sector traditionally dominated by private enterprise and leaving an indelible impact on the nation's healthcare system.

Shaping Access, Pricing, and Expectations

Medicare and Medicaid not only expanded the reach of healthcare in America but also fundamentally altered the dynamics of access, pricing, and public expectations. These programs introduced new paradigms of who could receive care, at what cost, and under what conditions, effectively reshaping the healthcare marketplace and the social contract between citizens and the state. While their implementation addressed glaring inequities, it also gave rise to complexities that continue to challenge policymakers, providers, and patients alike.

Access to healthcare, which had long been dictated by socioeconomic status, underwent a seismic shift with the advent of these programs. Medicare extended coverage to the elderly, a population disproportionately affected by chronic illnesses and limited incomes, while Medicaid targeted society's most vulnerable groups. These initiatives carved out a space for government as a guarantor of healthcare for specific populations, fostering an expectation that certain needs would be met irrespective of an individual's ability to pay. For the first time, millions of Americans who had been sidelined by the private insurance market—whether due to age, poverty, or pre-existing conditions—gained a foothold in the healthcare system. This newfound access, however, also exposed the limitations of supply: a surge in demand overwhelmed existing facilities, prompting expansions in hospital infrastructure and workforce training but also creating bottlenecks that underscored the fragility of the system.

In tandem with expanding access, Medicare and Medicaid exerted profound influence on healthcare pricing. The fee-for-service reimbursement model adopted by Medicare, which incentivized providers to bill for each individual service rendered, fueled an era of unprecedented medical spending. While this approach initially spurred innovations and expanded service offerings, it also entrenched inefficiencies and escalated costs. Providers, aware of guaranteed government reimbursement, had little incentive to control prices, leading to a proliferation of high-cost procedures and technologies. Medicaid, with its reliance on state-negotiated rates, introduced additional complexity. States frequently set reimbursement rates below market levels to control costs, which in turn discouraged provider participation and created disparities in care availability. The dual pressures of increasing demand and spiraling costs laid bare the inherent tensions in attempting to balance universal access with fiscal sustainability.

These programs also redefined public expectations of the healthcare system. Before their implementation, healthcare was largely seen as a privilege tied to employment or personal wealth. Medicare and Medicaid reframed it as a right for certain groups, embedding the notion that government bears some responsibility for ensuring basic health needs are met. This shift in expectations extended beyond the direct beneficiaries of these programs. Employers, insurers, and even private citizens began to view healthcare through a new lens, questioning why similar guarantees were not extended universally. The result was a growing public appetite for broader reforms, coupled with an increasing dissatisfaction with the system's inequities.

Yet, these changing expectations also revealed fault lines in the system's design. While Medicare and Medicaid brought millions into the fold, they left significant gaps in coverage and created a tiered system of care. Medicaid recipients often faced stigma and lower quality services compared to their Medicare counterparts, and the reliance on state administration perpetuated regional inequities. Moreover, the programs' initial structures did little to address the underlying drivers of poor health outcomes, such as socioeconomic disparities and systemic racism, which continued to limit access and quality for marginalized populations.

The interplay between access, pricing, and expectations catalyzed by Medicare and Medicaid has had enduring consequences. These programs, while groundbreaking in their scope, also exposed the paradoxes inherent in a hybrid healthcare system that straddles public and private interests. They demonstrated the potential for government to act as a corrective force in a market-driven landscape but also highlighted the constraints imposed by political compromise and economic realities. Over time, the growing complexity of managing costs and meeting expectations has necessitated an ongoing cycle of reforms, each grappling with the legacy of these foundational programs. Their impact, both as a promise fulfilled and a challenge left unresolved, remains at the heart of the American healthcare debate.

POLITICAL BATTLES AND IDEOLOGICAL DIVIDES

The creation of Medicare and Medicaid was not merely a legislative victory; it was a fiercely contested battle that exposed the deep ideological divides surrounding the role of government in healthcare. These programs were born out of an era marked by political maneuvering, philosophical clashes, and intense lobbying. The debates that preceded their passage—and the controversies that have persisted in their implementation—underscore the fundamentally polarized nature of American attitudes toward state involvement in public welfare.

At the heart of the political battles over Medicare and Medicaid was a broader ideological tension between collectivism and individualism. Proponents of the programs, largely led by Democrats under President Lyndon B. Johnson's Great Society vision, framed healthcare as a moral obligation of a modern state. They argued that a wealthy and industrialized nation had a duty to protect its most vulnerable citizens—whether the elderly, the disabled, or the poor—from the devastating consequences of unaffordable medical care. Medicare was pitched as a safeguard for dignity in old age, while Medicaid promised to extend a safety net for those left behind by the private insurance market. These arguments appealed to a growing public consciousness about inequality and the belief that government could and should act as a counterweight to the market's indifference to human suffering.

Opposition to the programs, however, was vehement and multifaceted. Conservative lawmakers and industry groups warned that federal involvement in healthcare would be a slippery slope toward socialism, eroding personal freedoms and fostering dependency on government aid. Private insurers and medical associations, particularly the American Medical Association (AMA), waged aggressive campaigns against Medicare, portraying it as a direct threat to the autonomy of physicians and the sanctity of the doctor-patient relationship. The AMA's "Operation Coffee Cup" campaign, for instance, mobilized physicians and community leaders to decry Medicare as an encroachment on private enterprise, often invoking Cold War fears of centralized control. This ideological resistance tapped into a deep-seated skepticism about federal overreach, a sentiment that resonated with a significant segment of the American populace.

The legislative process itself reflected these divides, with compromises shaping the programs into their eventual forms. Medicare, initially envisioned as a universal program for all citizens, was narrowed to focus solely on seniors and later expanded to include the disabled and those with end-stage renal disease. Medicaid, meanwhile, was designed as a federal-state partnership, a structure that allowed states significant latitude in determining eligibility and benefits. These compromises were necessary to secure bipartisan support, but they also embedded structural weaknesses that have perpetuated inequalities and inefficiencies. For example, Medicaid's reliance on state administration has resulted in vast disparities in access and quality of care across states, while Medicare's fee-for-service model laid the groundwork for cost inflation.

Even after their passage, Medicare and Medicaid remained battlegrounds for ideological conflict. In the decades that followed, successive administrations have sought to reshape or undermine these programs according to their political priorities. Conservative efforts to curtail Medicaid through block grants or work requirements have clashed with progressive attempts to expand its coverage. Medicare, too, has been a frequent target of reform, with debates over privatization, prescription drug benefits, and the rise of Medicare Advantage plans reflecting ongoing tensions about the balance between public oversight and private competition. These conflicts have not only influenced policy but also shaped public perceptions, reinforcing the narrative that healthcare is an inherently contentious and political issue in the United States.

The enduring ideological divides over Medicare and Medicaid highlight the challenges of reconciling competing visions for the future of healthcare. For some, these programs represent the first steps toward a more equitable and universal system; for others, they symbolize the dangers of government intervention in a domain best left to market forces. This polarization has limited the scope of reform, ensuring that Medicare and Medicaid remain both indispensable pillars of the healthcare system and perennial sources of political controversy. Their history serves as a stark reminder that the fight over healthcare is not just about policy but about the values and identities that define America itself.

UNINTENDED CONSEQUENCES

The introduction of Medicare and Medicaid, despite their noble intentions, gave rise to a series of unintended consequences that have had lasting implications for the U.S. healthcare system. These programs were designed to increase access to care for vulnerable populations, but their implementation inadvertently reshaped the dynamics of the healthcare market in ways that were not fully anticipated. From cost inflation to the fragmentation of care, the impact of these programs has been profound and often contradictory.

One of the most significant unintended consequences was the rapid rise in healthcare costs. Medicare and Medicaid were designed to protect the elderly, the poor, and the disabled from the financial ruin of medical bills. However, the sheer size and scope of these programs created a powerful demand for healthcare services, driving up overall expenditures. The fee-for-service model of Medicare, in particular, incentivized the provision of more services rather than the efficiency or quality of care. Physicians and hospitals were reimbursed for the volume of care they provided, regardless of outcomes, which led to an increase in unnecessary procedures and tests. This model, while initially beneficial in ensuring access, ultimately contributed to the spiraling costs of healthcare that are now a central challenge of the American system.

Medicaid, with its federal-state partnership, experienced its own set of challenges. The flexibility granted to states in administering the program led to significant disparities in coverage, care quality, and eligibility criteria. Some states were more generous with benefits, while others sought to limit access through restrictive eligibility requirements or low reimbursement rates for providers. These inconsistencies created a patchwork system that left many low-income individuals without adequate care or forced them into overcrowded, underfunded healthcare facilities. The disparity in Medicaid expansion following the Affordable Care Act, where some states opted out of Medicaid expansion altogether, further deepened these inequalities, leaving millions of Americans without the coverage they needed.

Another unintended consequence was the growth of private sector involvement in what had originally been envisioned as a government-provided safety net. As the demand for healthcare grew, private insurance companies saw opportunities to offer supplemental plans, often targeting the Medicare population through Medicare Advantage plans. While these private plans promised more benefits and more choice, they also introduced new layers of complexity and profit motives into a system that had previously been based on public provision. The rise of private insurers within Medicare has been criticized for diverting resources away from the public system and driving up overall costs. These plans, which are often marketed to seniors, have been criticized for misleading advertising and often provide limited care options compared to traditional Medicare.

The growth of Medicaid managed care was another unintended consequence of the program's expansion. In an effort to control costs, many states turned to private managed care organizations to oversee Medicaid beneficiaries' care. While these organizations were meant to streamline care and reduce costs, they also led to fragmentation. Beneficiaries often found themselves navigating a labyrinth of different insurers and providers, which created barriers to accessing care. Moreover, the cost-cutting measures of managed care often led to reduced provider reimbursements, causing many physicians to opt out of Medicaid altogether. This, in turn, limited access to care for millions of Medicaid beneficiaries, particularly in rural or underserved areas.

On a broader scale, the rise of Medicare and Medicaid also exacerbated the growing dependence on insurance as the primary mechanism for accessing healthcare. While the programs were designed to provide coverage for those who could not afford it, they also reinforced the idea that healthcare is a commodity best delivered through third-party insurance. This model, rather than fostering a more holistic or preventative approach to health, contributed to a focus on episodic, reactive care. As insurance companies, both public and private, became the dominant players in the healthcare system, the focus shifted away from addressing the root causes of health disparities and toward managing the financial risks associated with illness.

Moreover, the sheer scale of Medicare and Medicaid introduced a level of bureaucracy and administrative complexity that was not foreseen. Both programs, with their different rules, regulations, and procedures, required a vast administrative apparatus to manage claims, ensure compliance, and track reimbursements. This bureaucracy not only added significant costs to the system but also created barriers to care. Providers faced mountains of paperwork and delays in reimbursement, while patients were often left navigating a maze of eligibility rules, co-pays, and deductibles. The inefficiency and opacity of these systems have led to frustration among both healthcare providers and recipients, contributing to a sense of alienation and dissatisfaction with the system as a whole.

Finally, the creation of Medicare and Medicaid, while intended to reduce the burden of healthcare costs for vulnerable populations, also inadvertently entrenched healthcare as a highly fragmented and market-driven system. The fact that private insurance, managed care organizations, and public programs operate in parallel, with little coordination between them, has resulted in inefficiencies and confusion. This fragmentation has left millions of Americans caught in a system that is often difficult to navigate and, in many cases, doesn't provide the care they need when they need it most.

In sum, while Medicare and Medicaid were instrumental in expanding access to care for millions of Americans, the unintended consequences of these programs highlight the complexities and challenges inherent in any large-scale government intervention in the healthcare market. From rising costs to systemic inefficiencies, these programs have shaped the healthcare landscape in ways that continue to affect policy debates today. The lessons of these unintended consequences underscore the need for thoughtful reform and a deeper understanding of how government programs interact with the broader market forces that govern healthcare delivery.

Legacy and Contemporary Relevance

The legacy of Medicare and Medicaid is deeply intertwined with the contemporary structure of the U.S. healthcare system, providing a foundational understanding of how public programs interact with private forces and the broader economy. Over half a century after their creation, these programs continue to shape healthcare access, quality, and cost, while also influencing ongoing debates about health policy. Their legacy is a complex one—marked by both significant achievements and enduring challenges. The ongoing relevance of these programs lies in the persistent gaps they have both revealed and exacerbated, offering critical lessons for future policy decisions.

Medicare and Medicaid's legacy is especially pronounced in their role as pivotal markers in the ongoing tension between public and private sectors in U.S.

healthcare. These programs have offered millions of Americans—especially seniors, low-income individuals, and the disabled—access to essential healthcare services. For these groups, Medicare and Medicaid have been life-changing. However, the legacy is not without its flaws. The initial promise of universal care for vulnerable populations has not always been fully realized, and the way these programs have evolved has sometimes left them vulnerable to inefficiencies, political manipulation, and corporate entanglements.

The shift from a charitable, community-based care model to one dominated by private entities has profound implications for both policy and public opinion. As Medicare and Medicaid became more entwined with the for-profit healthcare industry, new dynamics emerged. Private insurers began playing a greater role, especially within Medicare through Medicare Advantage plans, which have expanded dramatically in recent years. These plans, while offering some advantages, such as additional benefits and flexibility, also illustrate a broader trend: the privatization of public programs. The expansion of private entities in these public programs has resulted in an increasingly fragmented system, where the interests of profit-driven corporations often seem at odds with the broader public interest.

Furthermore, Medicare and Medicaid's legacy can be seen in the current state of healthcare disparities. Despite the remarkable progress made in expanding access to care for historically underserved populations, the gap in health outcomes between the rich and poor, between racial and ethnic groups, and between urban and rural areas remains striking. While the Affordable Care Act (ACA) made strides in reducing the uninsured rate and expanding Medicaid, millions of Americans are still left without adequate care, particularly in states that chose not to expand Medicaid. The fragmentation of care, a direct consequence of the patchwork nature of Medicare and Medicaid, continues to leave many without timely access to services, especially in underserved regions or among those without supplemental insurance.

The rising cost of healthcare remains perhaps the most enduring and controversial consequence of Medicare and Medicaid. These programs were originally designed to alleviate the financial burden of care for vulnerable populations, but their implementation has inadvertently contributed to the broader inflation of healthcare costs in the U.S. The fee-for-service model of Medicare, for example, encouraged a volume-based approach to care, where the more tests, procedures, and treatments performed, the greater the reimbursement. This model, although intended to expand access to care, helped establish the fee-for-service paradigm that drives up the cost of healthcare for everyone, not just those relying on government programs. Similarly, Medicaid's expansion, while essential for providing coverage to low-income individuals, also has contributed to cost pressures in state budgets, particularly in states with high levels of Medicaid enrollment.

Despite these challenges, the programs continue to be a cornerstone of the U.S. healthcare system, especially in a nation where healthcare access remains a deeply contentious issue. Medicare, in particular, has come to symbolize the ongoing struggle over healthcare reform in America. As the baby boomer generation continues to age, the number of Medicare beneficiaries will rise significantly, placing further strain on the program's funding and the broader healthcare system. The looming financial challenges faced by Medicare and Medicaid require a reckoning about the sustainability of these programs in their current form and the need for reform.

In contemporary discussions, the legacy of these programs also plays a significant role in the political and ideological divides over healthcare reform. For some, Medicare and Medicaid are seen as essential programs that protect vulnerable populations and provide a model for universal care. For others, these programs represent the failure of government intervention in the market and a drain on national resources. The debate over Medicare for All, for instance, often pits advocates for a single-payer system against those who argue for the preservation of private insurance and market-driven healthcare. The legacy of Medicare and Medicaid thus continues to fuel these debates, as Americans continue to grapple with the best way to provide affordable, high-quality healthcare to all.

The contemporary relevance of Medicare and Medicaid also lies in the lessons they provide for future healthcare reform. As policymakers confront rising healthcare costs, aging populations, and growing health inequities, the experience of Medicare and Medicaid offers important guidance. It underscores the need for comprehensive, systemic reform that accounts for both the needs of vulnerable populations and the constraints imposed by market forces. It also highlights the importance of addressing not just access to care, but the quality of that care and its cost-effectiveness. Moreover, as technology continues to reshape healthcare delivery, the legacy of Medicare and Medicaid will be critical in shaping the integration of new technologies, such as telemedicine, into these programs in a way that benefits all stakeholders without exacerbating inequalities.

The legacy of Medicare and Medicaid is a testament to both the promise and limitations of government intervention in healthcare. While these programs have provided essential services to millions and continue to be a lifeline for many, their evolution has exposed deep challenges and contradictions within the U.S. healthcare system. Their contemporary relevance is undeniable, as the issues they have raised—cost, equity, quality, and sustainability—remain central to the ongoing debates over the future of healthcare in America. Understanding the legacy of Medicare and Medicaid is essential for anyone seeking to navigate the complex landscape of U.S. healthcare policy and reform, offering crucial insights into both the successes and the failures of the system.

PARADIGM SHIFTS AND PERSISTENT CHALLENGES

Over the decades, Medicare and Medicaid have catalyzed significant paradigm shifts in American healthcare, but they have also revealed persistent challenges that continue to shape the national discourse on access, quality, and equity. These programs, conceived as a safety net for the most vulnerable, have undergone transformative changes, influencing not only who receives care but also how care is delivered and funded. The shifts they initiated reflect broader societal changes, including the increasing commodification of health, the growing influence of technology, and the enduring tension between public welfare and private enterprise. Yet, for all the progress achieved, their evolution underscores challenges that remain unresolved, perpetuating disparities and raising critical questions about the future of U.S. healthcare.

One of the most profound paradigm shifts brought about by Medicare and Medicaid was the normalization of government involvement in healthcare. Prior to their establishment, the role of the state in ensuring access to medical care was minimal, leaving healthcare largely in the hands of private practitioners, hospitals, and charities. The introduction of these programs marked a turning point, signaling a federal commitment to addressing the healthcare needs of the elderly, the poor, and the disabled. This shift not only expanded access but also set a precedent for subsequent reforms, such as the Affordable Care Act, which sought to further broaden the safety net. However, it also sparked enduring ideological battles over the extent to which government should intervene in what many believe should remain a market-driven industry.

Another critical transformation has been the impact of Medicare and Medicaid on healthcare delivery systems. These programs have been instrumental in driving the consolidation of hospitals and the proliferation of managed care models. Initially designed to reimburse providers for services rendered, Medicare and Medicaid inadvertently incentivized the growth of large healthcare systems capable of navigating the complex requirements of federal funding. This consolidation has had mixed consequences: while it has streamlined some aspects of care delivery, it has also contributed to rising costs and the monopolization of healthcare markets. Managed care, particularly through Medicaid and Medicare Advantage, introduced new efficiencies but also raised concerns about access restrictions and the prioritization of cost savings over patient outcomes.

Technology has also played a significant role in shaping the evolution of these programs, ushering in a new era of data-driven healthcare. Medicare, for instance, has embraced value-based payment models that rely on electronic health records and performance metrics to reward providers for improving patient outcomes. Telemedicine, once a niche service, has become a critical component of care delivery, especially for Medicaid beneficiaries in rural or underserved areas. These technological advancements hold great promise for enhancing efficiency and access, but they also highlight persistent challenges. Disparities in digital literacy and access to technology can exacerbate inequalities, particularly among the populations these programs are designed to serve. Additionally, the reliance on data-driven models raises ethical questions about patient privacy and the potential for algorithmic biases in care decisions.

Despite these paradigm shifts, persistent challenges remain, particularly in the realm of equity. Medicare and Medicaid, while expansive, are not universal. Eligibility criteria and funding structures vary widely, leaving significant gaps in coverage. Medicaid, for instance, is administered at the state level, leading to a patchwork of programs with varying benefits and eligibility requirements. States that have opted not to expand Medicaid under the Affordable Care Act have created a coverage gap for low-income individuals who earn too much to qualify for traditional Medicaid but too little to afford private insurance. Similarly, Medicare's reliance on supplemental insurance to cover out-of-pocket costs leaves many beneficiaries exposed to financial hardship, undermining the program's goal of providing comprehensive care.

Cost remains another enduring challenge. Medicare and Medicaid collectively account for a significant portion of federal and state budgets, and their expenditures are projected to grow as the population ages and healthcare costs rise. Efforts to contain costs have often come at the expense of providers and beneficiaries. Reimbursement rates for Medicaid are notoriously low, discouraging many physicians from accepting Medicaid patients and limiting access to care. Medicare faces similar pressures, with debates over the program's solvency leading to proposals that would shift more costs onto beneficiaries or reduce payments to providers. These financial pressures not only threaten the sustainability of these programs but also highlight the broader challenge of balancing cost control with the need to ensure equitable access to high-quality care.

The evolving healthcare landscape also underscores the limitations of incremental reform in addressing systemic issues. Medicare and Medicaid, while transformative, were designed as targeted solutions rather than comprehensive reforms. As a result, they coexist with a fragmented system that includes employer-sponsored insurance, private plans, and the uninsured. This fragmentation perpetuates inefficiencies and inequities, creating a system that is both the most expensive in the world and one that delivers uneven outcomes. The ongoing reliance on incremental changes, such as adjustments to reimbursement models or eligibility criteria, reflects the political and ideological divisions that have stymied efforts to enact more sweeping reforms, such as single-payer healthcare.

In examining the paradigm shifts and persistent challenges associated with Medicare and Medicaid, it becomes clear that these programs are both a reflection of and a response to the broader dynamics of American society. They have transformed the healthcare system in profound ways, expanding access and driving innovation, but they have also exposed and, in some cases, exacerbated underlying inequities and inefficiencies. As the nation continues to grapple with the complexities of healthcare reform, the legacy of Medicare and Medicaid offers valuable lessons about the potential and the limits of government intervention in addressing one of the most pressing issues of our time. These programs serve as a reminder that while progress is possible, the path to a more equitable and sustainable healthcare system requires not just incremental adjustments but a willingness to confront the systemic barriers that hinder meaningful change.

CHAPTER 3: THE FREE MARKET TAKES OVER

The transformation of healthcare into a commodity reflects the deep entanglement of medicine and market forces in the United States. This shift was neither inevitable nor sudden; it was the result of deliberate decisions, shaped by historical context, economic imperatives, and cultural values that prioritized individualism and competition. Essentially lies a fundamental question: what happens when the provision of care, a deeply human necessity, is aligned with the mechanisms of profit and loss? The answer, as the United States demonstrates, is a system that is as innovative as it is unequal.

In the early days of American healthcare, the idea of medicine as a public good was more pronounced. Hospitals were places of charity, often run by religious institutions or supported by community funds, serving those in desperate need of care. Physicians operated as independent professionals, providing services on a fee-for-service basis, guided as much by social obligation as by financial reward. However, as the country grew, so did the pressures of modernization. The industrial revolution introduced new technologies, medical advancements, and demographic shifts that demanded a more organized approach to healthcare delivery. These pressures planted the seeds for a transition, one that would redefine the relationship between medicine and the marketplace.

By the mid-20th century, the alignment of healthcare with capitalist principles began to take shape. Two key forces accelerated this process. First, the introduction of employer-sponsored health insurance during World War II created a pathway for private markets to dominate healthcare financing. Originally a workaround to government-imposed wage controls, employer-sponsored insurance became a cornerstone of the system, tethering access to healthcare to one's place of employment. Second, the rapid advances in medical technology and pharmaceuticals brought with them enormous costs, necessitating systems that could manage and monetize the delivery of care. The convergence of these factors signaled a profound shift: the dawn of healthcare as a business.

This evolution was underpinned by a philosophical shift that saw healthcare less as a universal right and more as an economic good. Free-market principles, long heralded as engines of innovation and efficiency, found fertile ground in the healthcare sector. The industry became a natural site for market expansion, driven by the promise of technological progress and the allure of financial gain. Yet, as healthcare became increasingly enmeshed in the logic of capitalism, new tensions emerged. The incentives that spurred innovation also created barriers to access, transforming the act of receiving care into a transactional experience. For those with resources, the system offered world-class treatments and cutting-edge technologies. For others, it became a labyrinth of costs, exclusions, and unmet needs.

At the heart of this transition lies a paradox. The same forces that enabled the United States to lead the world in medical breakthroughs have also made it a global outlier in healthcare inequality. By intertwining medicine with the market, the country has cultivated a system that thrives on its ability to generate profit, often at the expense of equity and simplicity. Understanding how and why this happened is essential to grasping the broader dynamics of the American healthcare system—a system that has come to reflect the very contradictions of the society it serves.

THE RISE OF EMPLOYER-SPONSORED INSURANCE

The emergence of employer-sponsored insurance in the United States was not the result of careful planning or visionary policy. Instead, it was a historical accident, born out of economic necessity and political compromise during a time of national crisis. Yet, this development would fundamentally shape the trajectory of American healthcare, embedding private insurance into the very fabric of the system and creating a framework that persists to this day.

During World War II, the U.S. government implemented wage controls to curb inflation and stabilize the economy. Employers, unable to compete for workers through higher salaries, turned to alternative forms of compensation. Health insurance, previously a fringe benefit offered by only a few forward-thinking companies, became an attractive tool for recruitment and retention. This practice gained further traction when the federal government ruled that employer contributions to health insurance would be tax-exempt, effectively incentivizing businesses to adopt the model. What began as a temporary workaround to wartime restrictions quickly evolved into a defining feature of the American healthcare system.

The postwar economic boom solidified this arrangement. As industries flourished and unions gained strength, collective bargaining increasingly focused on securing robust health benefits. Employers, eager to attract skilled labor and maintain workforce stability, embraced the model, and health insurance became a standard part of employment packages. For workers, this represented a significant improvement in access to healthcare, particularly as medical advancements made care more effective—and more expensive. But this system, deeply reliant on private markets and tied to employment, also set the stage for the inequities and inefficiencies that would later define American healthcare.

The employer-sponsored model effectively created a two-tiered system. Those with stable jobs in industries that offered generous benefits enjoyed access to a growing array of medical services, while others—unemployed, self-employed, or working in sectors without such benefits—were left to fend for themselves. This division highlighted an underlying assumption of the system: healthcare was not a universal right but a benefit earned through participation in the labor market. As a result, access to care became inherently tied to one's economic status, reinforcing broader social inequalities.

Moreover, this approach entrenched the dominance of private insurance companies. As employers sought to manage costs and expand coverage options, insurers became powerful intermediaries, shaping the rules of the game. They negotiated prices with hospitals, dictated reimbursement policies for physicians, and determined which treatments would be covered. Over time, the interests of these companies increasingly aligned with profit maximization, introducing complexities and administrative burdens that would ripple through the entire system. The relationship between employers, insurers, and providers created a healthcare ecosystem that prioritized the financial bottom line as much as—or more than—the needs of patients.

The rise of employer-sponsored insurance also carried unintended consequences for the broader healthcare landscape. It fragmented the system, creating silos of coverage that made it difficult to achieve universal access or negotiate consistent pricing. Unlike countries where centralized systems allowed for coordinated care and cost control, the U.S. developed a patchwork model, leaving millions uninsured or underinsured. Furthermore, as healthcare costs escalated in subsequent decades, the employer-sponsored model came under increasing strain, with small businesses and low-wage industries struggling to provide adequate coverage.

This system's endurance reflects both its strengths and its flaws. On one hand, it has enabled millions of Americans to access high-quality care through their employment. On the other, it has left the system vulnerable to economic shocks, such as recessions, that disrupt job-based coverage. By embedding healthcare so deeply into the employer-employee relationship, the U.S. created a uniquely privatized system that reinforces market-driven principles while amplifying social disparities—a dynamic that continues to define the nation's healthcare debates.

Insurance Giants and the Birth of an Industry

The rise of private insurance giants was a pivotal moment in the evolution of the American healthcare system, transforming it from a fragmented collection of localized practices into a sprawling industry defined by corporate dominance and financial complexity. While employer-sponsored insurance laid the groundwork for broader coverage, the emergence of powerful insurance companies institutionalized a profit-driven framework that would dictate the priorities and operations of U.S. healthcare for decades to come.

In the mid-20th century, as employer-based health benefits became widespread, insurers began to consolidate their influence. Companies like Blue Cross and Blue Shield, originally non-profit entities established to provide affordable access to healthcare, were among the first to scale their operations. Initially, their mission was rooted in community-based coverage, with premiums calculated to ensure broad accessibility rather than maximize revenue. However, as the demand for health insurance surged, these organizations faced mounting competition from private, for-profit insurers eager to capitalize on a burgeoning market.

The shift from community-focused to profit-oriented insurance represented a profound departure from the original ethos of healthcare as a public good. For-profit insurers introduced risk-based pricing, a model in which premiums were tailored to individual health profiles, employment sectors, and geographic regions. While this approach allowed for competitive pricing in some segments, it also systematically excluded high-risk individuals and marginalized communities. Those with pre-existing conditions, chronic illnesses, or limited economic means often found themselves unable to afford coverage, exacerbating inequalities that persist to this day.

As competition intensified, insurance companies began leveraging their growing economic power to reshape the healthcare landscape. They negotiated with hospitals and physicians to establish network contracts, effectively creating hierarchies of care providers. In exchange for funneling patients to specific hospitals or practices, insurers demanded discounted rates, a practice that reinforced the economic clout of larger, urban healthcare providers while marginalizing smaller, rural institutions. Over time, this dynamic contributed to the consolidation of healthcare delivery, as hospitals merged or were acquired to strengthen their negotiating positions.

The growth of the insurance industry also introduced new layers of bureaucracy into healthcare. Administrative processes such as claims management, pre-authorization requirements, and utilization reviews became standard practices, ostensibly aimed at controlling costs and preventing unnecessary procedures. However, these measures often placed significant burdens on patients and providers alike. Physicians, once the central figures in determining care, found their decisions increasingly subject to approval by insurance administrators, while patients faced bewildering arrays of rules, coverage limitations, and out-of-pocket expenses. The result was a system that prioritized cost containment for insurers but frequently undermined the quality and accessibility of care for individuals.

One of the defining features of the insurance industry's dominance was its ability to shape policy through lobbying and political influence. By the late 20th century, health insurers had become some of the most powerful entities in Washington, funneling billions of dollars into campaign contributions and advocacy efforts. Their lobbying clout ensured that legislative reforms—whether designed to expand access, regulate pricing, or curb industry abuses—were often diluted or structured to protect their interests. The Affordable Care Act of 2010, for example, mandated that individuals obtain health insurance but preserved the role of private insurers as primary intermediaries, guaranteeing them a steady flow of customers while limiting broader systemic reforms.

The consolidation of power within the insurance industry also set the stage for escalating healthcare costs. With limited regulation over premium pricing and significant market leverage, insurers could pass rising medical expenses onto consumers and employers. Meanwhile, their profit motives drove the proliferation of high-deductible plans, narrow provider networks, and increased cost-sharing mechanisms, shifting more financial risk onto patients. As a result, many Americans found themselves insured in name but financially exposed in practice, unable to afford necessary care despite holding coverage.

The rise of insurance giants marked the transformation of American healthcare into a market-driven juggernaut, where the imperatives of profit frequently clashed with the needs of patients. While these companies played a critical role in expanding access and organizing a fragmented system, they also entrenched systemic inefficiencies and inequities. Today, the legacy of this era is evident in the enduring tension between private profit and public good—a dynamic that continues to fuel debates over the future of U.S. healthcare.

THE MEDICAL-INDUSTRIAL COMPLEX

The term *medical-industrial complex* aptly captures the sprawling web of corporations, providers, and intermediaries that coalesced in the late 20th century, transforming American healthcare into a market-driven enterprise of staggering complexity and scale. Unlike its origins as a decentralized network of practitioners and small-scale institutions, the U.S. healthcare system became increasingly dominated by a coalition of interests: hospital chains, pharmaceutical manufacturers, medical device companies, and insurers. These stakeholders, while ostensibly aligned around the delivery of care, were often united more by financial interests than by a shared commitment to improving patient outcomes.

The seeds of the medical-industrial complex were sown in the post-World War II era, as advances in medical technology and treatments spurred rapid growth in healthcare expenditures. By the 1960s, government programs like Medicare and Medicaid further accelerated this trend by injecting billions of dollars into the system, creating an environment ripe for profit-seeking. As public funding expanded, so too did the opportunities for private-sector players to extract value at every stage of care delivery. This confluence of public investment and private enterprise cemented healthcare as one of the most lucrative industries in the United States.

Hospitals, once community-based institutions devoted to charitable care, evolved into corporate entities seeking to maximize revenue streams. For-profit hospital chains proliferated, consolidating smaller facilities into regional systems that wielded considerable market power. These systems aggressively pursued capital investments in advanced diagnostic tools, surgical suites, and specialty care centers, often financed by issuing debt or seeking private equity backing. The result was a sharp escalation in the cost of care, as the pursuit of high-margin services overshadowed the delivery of routine or preventive care.

Pharmaceutical companies, meanwhile, emerged as dominant players within the medical-industrial complex. The development of life-saving drugs and groundbreaking therapies generated unprecedented profits, but it also underscored the system's profit-first ethos. By the 1980s, the industry had mastered the art of marketing, employing aggressive direct-to-consumer advertising and leveraging physician incentives to promote high-cost medications over more affordable alternatives. Pricing strategies, particularly for patented drugs, often bore little relation to production costs, with companies citing the need to recoup research and development expenses as justification for exorbitant prices. This argument, while partially valid, masked the reality of record-breaking profit margins and the systematic exploitation of a captive consumer base.

Medical device manufacturers followed a similar trajectory, focusing on innovation and marketing to capture market share. From artificial joints to implantable cardiac devices, the industry offered transformative technologies that improved countless lives. Yet, like their pharmaceutical counterparts, device makers were frequently criticized for prioritizing profitability over accessibility. High sticker prices, coupled with opaque contracting practices between manufacturers, hospitals, and insurers, ensured that even the most essential devices remained out of reach for many patients.

At the heart of the medical-industrial complex was a business model that thrived on inefficiency and fragmentation. Unlike other industries, where competition drives down costs and improves quality, healthcare's unique structure often rewarded waste. Hospitals and providers operated on fee-for-service models, incentivizing the volume of care rather than its value. Pharmaceutical and device companies exploited regulatory loopholes to extend patent protections, stymie generic competition, and inflate prices. Insurers, tasked with managing costs, added their own layers of bureaucracy, introducing administrative hurdles that often delayed or denied care. This mutually reinforcing cycle of profit-driven practices entrenched a system where financial gain frequently took precedence over patient welfare.

The influence of the medical-industrial complex extended far beyond the realm of care delivery, shaping public policy and societal perceptions of healthcare. Lobbying efforts by industry groups ensured that any significant reform would face stiff resistance. Attempts to regulate drug pricing, reduce administrative waste, or promote alternative payment models were often watered down or blocked entirely. Meanwhile, industry-funded advocacy campaigns framed the high costs of American healthcare as the inevitable byproduct of its quality and innovation, cultivating a narrative that stymied calls for systemic change.

For patients and providers alike, the consequences of this complex were profound. While technological advances and pharmaceutical breakthroughs offered hope and improved outcomes for many, they also exacerbated disparities in access and affordability. Millions of Americans found themselves caught in a system that could deliver miraculous cures for those who could pay, while leaving others to navigate insurmountable financial barriers. Providers, too, faced mounting pressures, as the demands of working within an increasingly corporatized system often clashed with their ethical obligations to prioritize patient care.

The rise of the medical-industrial complex represented a watershed moment in the evolution of U.S. healthcare, embedding market dynamics at its core. While this system fostered remarkable innovation and economic growth, it also entrenched inefficiencies, inequalities, and unsustainable cost trajectories. As the nation grapples with the challenges of reform, the medical-industrial complex looms large, a testament to the tension between the imperatives of profit and the ideals of care.

THE ROLE OF LEGISLATION IN CEMENTING PRIVATIZATION

The evolution of the U.S. healthcare system into a privatized, profit-oriented enterprise was not merely the result of market forces but was actively shaped by legislative decisions over decades. Laws and policies passed at both state and federal levels created the conditions for the privatization of care, solidifying the dominance of private entities and establishing healthcare as one of the most lucrative sectors of the American economy. While some legislative milestones aimed to improve access or efficiency, many inadvertently deepened the divide between those who benefited from the system and those who were left behind.

The Employee Retirement Income Security Act (ERISA) of 1974 exemplifies the ways in which legislation could empower private players while sidelining public oversight. Originally intended to protect employee benefits, ERISA had far-reaching implications for employer-sponsored health insurance. By preempting state laws that regulated health plans, ERISA allowed self-insured employers to escape certain state mandates, such as requirements to cover specific treatments. This not only gave large corporations significant leverage in shaping their healthcare offerings but also placed them beyond the reach of consumer protections enacted at the state level. The result was a patchwork system where the scope of benefits often depended on the employer's priorities rather than patient needs.

Another pivotal legislative development was the Health Maintenance Organization (HMO) Act of 1973. Championed as a solution to rising healthcare costs, the act encouraged the proliferation of HMOs by providing federal grants and loans for their establishment. These organizations were designed to deliver care more efficiently by managing costs and limiting unnecessary procedures. However, as private companies embraced the HMO model, its profit-driven implementation often led to restrictive practices, such as denying coverage for costly treatments or limiting patient choice in selecting providers. The focus shifted from quality care to cost containment, fueling widespread dissatisfaction and skepticism about managed care.

The 1980s ushered in a new era of deregulation under the Reagan administration, which significantly accelerated the privatization of healthcare. One of the most consequential changes came with the introduction of the Medicare Prospective Payment System (PPS) in 1983. This system replaced the traditional cost-based reimbursement model with fixed payments for hospital services based on diagnostic categories, or DRGs (Diagnosis-Related Groups). While intended to control Medicare spending, PPS inadvertently incentivized hospitals to maximize profits by focusing on high-revenue services and discharging patients more quickly. Private hospitals, in particular, seized the opportunity to optimize their revenue streams, often at the expense of comprehensive or preventive care.

Simultaneously, legislative changes opened the door for private insurers to play an increasingly central role in Medicare. The Balanced Budget Act of 1997, for instance, introduced Medicare Advantage (originally Medicare+Choice), allowing private insurance companies to offer Medicare plans. While proponents argued this would provide beneficiaries with more choices, critics pointed out that private plans often cherry-picked healthier patients, leaving traditional Medicare to cover sicker, costlier populations. Over time, Medicare Advantage grew into a dominant force, funneling billions of taxpayer dollars into private insurance companies while perpetuating disparities in care.

Pharmaceutical policy also played a critical role in cementing privatization, particularly with the passage of the Medicare Prescription Drug, Improvement, and Modernization Act of 2003. This legislation, which established Medicare Part D, outsourced the administration of prescription drug benefits to private insurers and explicitly prohibited Medicare from negotiating drug prices. This prohibition effectively handed pharmaceutical companies unparalleled pricing power, ensuring that the U.S. would continue to pay some of the highest drug prices in the world. The act epitomized the government's reliance on market-based solutions to expand access, even as these solutions deepened the system's inefficiencies and inequities.

Beyond healthcare-specific legislation, broader economic and regulatory policies also reinforced privatization. Antitrust enforcement in the healthcare sector, for instance, waned during critical periods, allowing hospital chains, insurance companies, and pharmaceutical firms to consolidate into powerful monopolies and oligopolies. Mergers and acquisitions became the norm, with lawmakers often framing consolidation as a pathway to efficiency and innovation. In practice, however, these mergers reduced competition, drove up costs, and limited consumer choice. The legislative environment thus created a paradox: while policymakers sought to foster competition, the system they built often entrenched monopolistic practices.

The Affordable Care Act (ACA) of 2010 offers a more recent example of legislation that, while expanding access, also entrenched privatization. The ACA's insurance marketplaces relied on private insurers to provide coverage, with subsidies to make plans more affordable. Although millions of Americans gained insurance through the ACA, the reliance on private markets preserved the profit motives of insurers, perpetuating many of the system's fundamental inefficiencies. Moreover, the Medicaid expansion under the ACA, while transformative for low-income populations in states that adopted it, often funneled funds through private managed care organizations, further embedding private interests in public healthcare programs.

Taken together, these legislative milestones illustrate how the U.S. healthcare system evolved into a privatized framework deeply intertwined with corporate power. Each law, whether explicitly designed to foster privatization or not, contributed to a system where private entities wield significant influence over access, pricing, and delivery of care. The role of government, rather than providing a counterbalance to market excesses, often facilitated the very conditions that allowed profit motives to dominate. By cementing privatization through policy, lawmakers ensured that the healthcare system would remain a reflection of broader American values—innovation, individualism, and, ultimately, inequality.

Profits Over Patients: The Consequences of Privatization

The privatization of healthcare in the United States, while championed as a means to foster efficiency, innovation, and consumer choice, has come at a profound cost to patients. The prioritization of profits over care has created a system that is not only fragmented and inequitable but one where the pursuit of financial gains often directly conflicts with the well-being of those it purports to serve. The consequences of this profit-driven ethos permeate every aspect of the system, from the delivery of care to its affordability and accessibility.

One of the most visible manifestations of privatization's consequences is the skyrocketing cost of care. The United States spends more on healthcare per capita than any other developed nation, yet outcomes such as life expectancy and chronic disease management lag behind those of countries with more publicly oriented systems. This disparity stems in part from the profit imperative driving up prices at every level of the system. Pharmaceutical companies, for instance, set exorbitant prices for life-saving drugs, often justifying their actions with the cost of research and development. Yet these prices frequently bear little relationship to actual R&D expenditures, with much of the revenue funneled into marketing campaigns, stock buybacks, and executive compensation.

Hospitals, too, have embraced a profit-maximizing approach, particularly as many have shifted from nonprofit to for-profit models or been absorbed into large health systems. These entities often focus on lucrative service lines such as cardiac and orthopedic care while cutting back on less profitable areas like mental health or rural outreach. The result is a landscape where access to certain types of care depends as much on geography and demographics as on medical need. Rural hospital closures, for example, have become an epidemic, leaving vast swathes of the country without critical healthcare infrastructure. This trend disproportionately affects low-income and elderly populations, who are left to navigate long distances for care or forgo treatment altogether.

The privatized insurance market further compounds these issues. Insurers, motivated by shareholder returns, deploy strategies designed to minimize payouts, such as narrow networks, high deductibles, and complex pre-authorization requirements. Patients often find themselves ensnared in a maze of bureaucracy, where accessing care becomes a battle of persistence and paperwork. Even for those with insurance, out-of-pocket costs can be debilitating. High premiums, co-pays, and unexpected medical bills contribute to medical debt being one of the leading causes of bankruptcy in the United States—a grim testament to a system that prioritizes financial metrics over human health.

Privatization's consequences extend beyond financial strain to the quality of care itself. The rise of for-profit entities has introduced incentives that can distort clinical decision-making, encouraging overutilization of profitable procedures while underemphasizing preventive care. Physicians often face pressures from administrators to meet revenue targets, subtly shifting their focus from patient-centered care to metrics that align with the bottom line. This dynamic erodes the trust that is foundational to the doctor-patient relationship and contributes to widespread dissatisfaction among both providers and patients.

Healthcare workers, who form the backbone of the system, bear the brunt of these distortions. Privatization has often translated into cost-cutting measures that lead to staff shortages, increased workloads, and burnout. Nurses, in particular, frequently find themselves stretched thin, juggling the demands of patient care with administrative tasks dictated by profit-driven metrics. This erosion of working conditions not only harms healthcare workers but also diminishes the quality of care patients receive, as overstressed staff struggle to maintain the standards of compassion and attention their roles demand.

The inequities entrenched by privatization are perhaps its most damning consequence. While the system works well for those who can afford its premiums and fees, it marginalizes vulnerable populations—low-income individuals, racial minorities, and the uninsured. These groups face systemic barriers to accessing care, from a lack of affordable insurance options to implicit biases within clinical settings. The privatized model, by design, caters to those with the means to pay, leaving the rest to rely on overstretched public systems, charity care, or nothing at all.

Privatization has also fostered a culture of short-term thinking, where immediate profits often take precedence over long-term public health. Investments in preventive care, health education, and community health initiatives are often sidelined in favor of services that generate immediate revenue. This neglect of prevention exacerbates health disparities and contributes to the chronic disease burden that strains the system as a whole. The COVID-19 pandemic starkly highlighted these vulnerabilities, exposing how profit-driven decision-making left the system ill-prepared to handle a large-scale public health crisis.

Yet, perhaps the most insidious consequence of privatization is its normalization of healthcare as a commodity rather than a right. In a profit-driven system, patients are redefined as consumers, and health becomes a transactional good. This shift has profound implications for societal values, fostering a mindset where access to care is viewed as a privilege rather than a collective responsibility. Such a perspective not only entrenches inequities but also limits the political will for transformative change, as those who benefit from the system's current structure resist reforms that might disrupt their advantages.

The consequences of privatization are neither accidental nor inevitable; they are the result of deliberate policy choices and systemic priorities. They reflect a healthcare system that operates less as a means of promoting public welfare and more as a vehicle for economic gain. While the U.S. model has undeniably fostered innovation and advanced medical science, its human cost raises urgent questions about the ethical and practical sustainability of prioritizing profits over patients. As the system continues to evolve, the challenge lies in finding a balance where the benefits of privatization do not come at the expense of those it was meant to serve.

Market Innovations and the Double-Edged Sword

The privatized nature of the U.S. healthcare system has undeniably spurred remarkable innovation, from groundbreaking pharmaceutical breakthroughs to cutting-edge medical technologies. These advancements reflect the powerful incentives embedded within a market-driven framework, where competition fosters creativity and investment in research and development. However, these same market forces often create a paradox: while driving progress, they can also exacerbate inequities and inefficiencies, leaving the system both a marvel of innovation and a source of profound frustration for many.

Pharmaceutical companies, for example, are among the most prominent beneficiaries of market incentives. The pursuit of profit has driven the development of life-saving medications, from antiretroviral drugs for HIV/AIDS to breakthrough treatments for cancer and rare genetic disorders. These achievements have transformed countless lives, demonstrating the capacity of privatized healthcare to deliver extraordinary results. Yet this progress often comes with a steep price tag. The market-driven approach encourages pharmaceutical firms to prioritize drugs with high profitability over those addressing less lucrative conditions, such as tropical diseases or preventive care solutions. Moreover, the practice of evergreening—making minor modifications to existing drugs to extend patent protections—has allowed companies to maintain monopolies, driving up costs and limiting access.

Medical technology has followed a similar trajectory. The United States leads the world in the development of advanced diagnostic tools, surgical techniques, and digital health platforms. Technologies like robotic surgery systems and personalized medicine have revolutionized patient care, offering precision and effectiveness unimaginable a few decades ago. Telemedicine, bolstered by the COVID-19 pandemic, has expanded access to care for many, particularly in underserved areas. Yet these innovations often reinforce the divide between those who can afford the latest technologies and those relegated to outdated or less effective treatments. The financial barriers to accessing these advancements mean that the benefits of innovation frequently accrue to wealthier populations, deepening existing disparities.

Market forces also influence how these innovations are integrated into the healthcare ecosystem. In a system driven by profits, providers and institutions are incentivized to adopt technologies and treatments that generate revenue, sometimes at the expense of clinical necessity. High-cost procedures or expensive imaging technologies may be overutilized, contributing to the system's inefficiencies. At the same time, innovations that could reduce costs or improve accessibility—such as generic drugs or community-based care models—often struggle to gain traction, as their financial rewards are less compelling within a profit-driven framework.

The insurance industry, too, has embraced innovation, albeit in ways that are often a double-edged sword for patients. Algorithms and data analytics have enabled insurers to better predict risks, design tailored policies, and streamline administrative processes. However, these same tools can be used to deny coverage, increase premiums, or restrict access to care through narrow networks. While insurers argue that these measures help control costs, the burden frequently falls on patients, who must navigate increasingly complex systems to receive care. The rise of value-based care models, which tie provider reimbursement to patient outcomes, exemplifies this tension. While these models aim to improve quality and efficiency, they also risk creating perverse incentives, such as avoiding high-risk patients who could negatively impact outcome metrics.

Startups and nontraditional players entering the healthcare market have further complicated the landscape. Companies like Amazon and Apple have ventured into healthcare, offering new approaches to consumer-centric care. These innovations promise to disrupt entrenched inefficiencies and bring fresh perspectives to longstanding challenges. Yet their focus on profitable niches, such as telehealth for well-insured populations or wearable health devices, raises questions about their ability—or willingness—to address the systemic issues affecting the uninsured and underinsured.

One of the most contentious aspects of market innovation lies in its impact on healthcare pricing. The absence of price regulation in the U.S. system has created an environment where the costs of drugs, procedures, and devices are often opaque and subject to significant markup. Hospitals, for instance, routinely charge widely varying prices for the same procedure, depending on a patient's insurance plan or lack thereof. While proponents argue that market-based pricing reflects the value of innovation and allows for reinvestment in future advancements, critics contend that this model places an undue financial burden on patients and undermines equitable access to care.

The role of government in this dynamic is both supportive and contradictory. Public funding through agencies like the National Institutes of Health (NIH) underpins much of the foundational research that private companies later commercialize. Yet, the profits from these innovations largely accrue to private entities, while taxpayers who funded the initial research often face high costs when accessing the resulting treatments. This public-private interplay highlights a key tension in the U.S. healthcare model: the reliance on public investment to fuel private profit.

Despite these challenges, the potential of market-driven innovation remains undeniable. The entrepreneurial spirit fostered by privatization has produced solutions to some of the most pressing medical challenges of our time. However, the system's failure to balance innovation with equity undermines its broader promise. The challenge moving forward is to harness the strengths of market forces while mitigating their excesses, ensuring that innovation serves the collective good rather than deepening divides.

Ultimately, the story of market innovation in U.S. healthcare is one of extraordinary achievements shadowed by persistent inequities. The system's ability to push the boundaries of what is medically possible is unparalleled, but its inability to ensure that these advancements benefit all Americans equally remains its greatest limitation. For the healthcare system to truly work for everyone, innovation must be coupled with reforms that prioritize access, affordability, and equity, ensuring that the benefits of progress are not confined to the privileged few.

The Insurance Industry's Dominance

The insurance industry occupies a central, inescapable role in the U.S. healthcare system, wielding unparalleled influence over how care is accessed, delivered, and paid for. What began as a pragmatic solution to spread financial risk and make healthcare affordable has evolved into an industry whose dominance often dictates not only patient outcomes but also the priorities of providers and policymakers. This transformation is emblematic of the privatized ethos driving American healthcare—a system where intermediaries profit from navigating the complex intersection of care and commerce.

At the heart of the insurance industry's power lies its role as the primary gatekeeper of care. Insurers determine which treatments, medications, and services are covered, imposing pre-authorization requirements and other restrictions that can delay or deny care. For patients, these decisions often mean navigating a labyrinth of bureaucratic processes to receive even basic treatment. While insurers argue that such measures are necessary to control costs and prevent unnecessary utilization, the reality for many patients is a system that feels opaque, adversarial, and indifferent to their immediate health needs.

This dominance is further reinforced by the industry's consolidation. Over the past few decades, mergers and acquisitions have left the insurance market in the hands of a few powerful players, such as UnitedHealth Group, Anthem, and Aetna. These corporations leverage their size to negotiate aggressively with providers, often dictating payment rates and coverage terms. While insurers tout their ability to reduce costs through economies of scale, the consolidation has also stifled competition, leaving consumers with limited choices and little leverage. In many regions, a single insurer holds a virtual monopoly, dictating terms not only to patients but also to hospitals and physicians.

One of the more insidious consequences of this consolidation is the rise of narrow networks—health plans that restrict patients to a limited set of providers. While marketed as a cost-saving measure, narrow networks often force patients to travel long distances, endure lengthy waits, or forgo care altogether when their preferred doctors or hospitals are out-of-network. The financial penalties for venturing outside these networks can be devastating, leaving patients to choose between crippling medical bills and inadequate care.

For providers, the insurance industry's dominance reshapes their priorities and practices. Physicians and hospitals increasingly find themselves constrained by insurers' payment models, which emphasize cost containment over patient-centered care. The rise of fee-for-service reimbursement—where providers are paid per procedure or visit—has incentivized quantity over quality, leading to the overutilization of certain tests and treatments while discouraging holistic, preventive approaches. Efforts to shift toward value-based care, where payments are tied to patient outcomes, have been met with mixed success, as the metrics used to define "value" often reflect insurers' priorities rather than patients' needs.

The administrative burden imposed by insurers further compounds these challenges. Physicians and hospitals must dedicate significant resources to complying with insurance requirements, from coding procedures to appealing denied claims. Studies have shown that U.S. healthcare providers spend far more on administrative overhead than their counterparts in other developed nations, with much of this expense driven by the complexity of navigating insurance systems. For smaller practices and rural hospitals, the financial strain of dealing with insurers can be existential, pushing many to close their doors or merge with larger entities.

Patients, too, bear the brunt of these dynamics. High-deductible health plans, increasingly common as employers seek to shift costs onto workers, leave many individuals and families facing significant out-of-pocket expenses before their insurance coverage even begins. The rise of coinsurance—a percentage of costs that patients must pay in addition to their premiums—further erodes the financial protection that insurance is supposed to provide. For those with chronic conditions or serious illnesses, these expenses can quickly spiral into unmanageable medical debt, undermining the very purpose of insurance.

The insurance industry's influence extends well beyond the confines of its direct interactions with patients and providers. Through extensive lobbying and campaign contributions, insurers shape the legislative and regulatory environment to their advantage. Their sway has been instrumental in preserving the fragmented, privatized structure of U.S. healthcare, resisting efforts to implement single-payer models or other reforms that might reduce their role. Even landmark legislation like the Affordable Care Act, which expanded coverage to millions, was heavily influenced by insurers' interests, incorporating provisions like the individual mandate to ensure a steady stream of enrollees while avoiding more disruptive reforms.

Critics of the insurance industry often point to its profit motives as a fundamental flaw in the system. Publicly traded insurers are accountable to shareholders, not patients, creating an inherent tension between maximizing profits and delivering affordable, high-quality care. The industry's defenders, however, argue that profit incentives drive efficiency and innovation, encouraging insurers to develop new models of care management and risk assessment. Yet even these innovations are frequently designed to benefit the bottom line rather than address systemic inequities or improve patient outcomes.

One of the most striking examples of this duality is the growth of Medicare Advantage plans—private insurance options for Medicare beneficiaries. These plans, which promise comprehensive coverage and lower out-of-pocket costs, have become immensely popular, enrolling nearly half of all Medicare recipients. However, critics argue that insurers have exploited the system by overbilling the government through practices like upcoding, where patients are classified as sicker than they are to receive higher payments. While Medicare Advantage plans illustrate how insurers can innovate within a public framework, they also highlight the challenges of balancing private profit with public accountability.

The insurance industry's dominance reflects the broader tensions within the U.S. healthcare system. It is both a product and a driver of privatization, shaping a system that prioritizes financial sustainability over universal access. While the industry has undoubtedly played a role in expanding coverage and managing risks, its influence often comes at the expense of transparency, equity, and patient trust. For meaningful reform to occur, the role of insurers must be reimagined, balancing their strengths with safeguards that prioritize the needs of patients over profits. Only then can the promise of insurance—to provide security and peace of mind—be fully realized in a system that works for all.

HEALTHCARE AS A MARKET COMMODITY

The transformation of healthcare into a market commodity marks one of the most profound shifts in the U.S. healthcare system's history. What was once considered a public good—a basic necessity for human dignity and survival—has become a product subject to the dynamics of supply and demand, competition, and consumer choice. This commodification has fundamentally reshaped how care is delivered, valued, and experienced, introducing efficiencies and innovations but also amplifying inequities and moral tensions.

In a market framework, healthcare providers, insurers, and pharmaceutical companies operate not as altruistic entities but as businesses driven by profit motives. Hospitals are no longer merely centers of healing; they are branded institutions competing for patients and prestige. Pharmaceutical firms prioritize blockbuster drugs with high profit margins over treatments for less common but equally debilitating conditions. Insurers, as intermediaries, thrive on complex financial arrangements that obscure the true costs of care. Even physicians, once regarded as autonomous caregivers, are often treated as units of productivity within larger systems, pressured to meet quotas and maximize revenue.

One of the defining features of healthcare as a commodity is the notion of consumer choice. Patients, rebranded as "healthcare consumers," are expected to navigate an increasingly complex marketplace, evaluating providers, treatments, and insurance plans based on price, quality, and convenience. In theory, this empowers individuals to take control of their health and incentivizes providers to compete on value. In practice, however, the opacity of pricing, variability in quality, and asymmetry of information often leave patients overwhelmed and disadvantaged. Few consumers, for example, can shop for an MRI or emergency surgery the way they might compare prices for a car or a vacation. The stakes are higher, the choices more constrained, and the consequences of misinformation far graver.

This commodification has also altered how value is perceived in healthcare. Instead of prioritizing outcomes like improved health or reduced suffering, value is increasingly measured in financial terms: revenue generated per patient, cost savings achieved through efficiency, or market share captured by a new treatment or facility. While these metrics are critical for the business sustainability of healthcare institutions, they often obscure the human dimension of care. The emphasis on profitability can lead to cost-cutting measures that compromise patient safety, such as understaffing, over-reliance on technology, or denying coverage for essential treatments deemed "non-cost-effective."

Healthcare's commodification extends beyond services to the very innovations that drive the field forward. Pharmaceutical breakthroughs, cutting-edge surgical techniques, and diagnostic technologies are celebrated not only for their clinical impact but also for their commercial success. Patents and intellectual property rights, while critical for incentivizing innovation, often result in monopolistic pricing that places life-saving treatments out of reach for many. The cost of insulin, for instance, has skyrocketed despite being an essential medication discovered over a century ago. The commodification of such advancements ensures their creators reap financial rewards, but it also entrenches disparities in access and outcomes.

The framing of healthcare as a market commodity is perhaps most starkly evident in the United States' pricing system. Unlike other developed nations, where governments play a central role in regulating healthcare costs, the U.S. system allows for significant price variability. The cost of a single procedure, such as a cesarean section, can vary dramatically depending on the hospital, the insurer, and the region. This variability reflects not only differences in quality or complexity but also the market power of providers and insurers, who negotiate prices behind closed doors. Patients, often unaware of these negotiations, bear the financial consequences, facing surprise medical bills and out-of-pocket expenses that defy any logical sense of value or fairness.

The commodification of healthcare also fuels broader societal inequities. Wealthier individuals and communities, with greater purchasing power, can access better providers, facilities, and treatments, while lower-income populations are relegated to underfunded clinics, overburdened hospitals, and limited options. This stratification is particularly evident in elective procedures, boutique healthcare services, and concierge medicine, where personalized, high-quality care is available to those who can afford it. For the rest, the commodification of healthcare often feels less like empowerment and more like exclusion.

Critics of healthcare commodification argue that it undermines the ethical foundations of medicine. The Hippocratic Oath, which binds physicians to prioritize patients' well-being, clashes with the profit-driven imperatives of a commodified system. When treatments are withheld due to cost, when billing departments dictate the scope of care, or when providers are incentivized to prioritize lucrative procedures over necessary ones, the moral compass of healthcare is skewed. Advocates for a more equitable system argue that healthcare should be recognized as a fundamental right rather than a commodity, with access determined by need rather than ability to pay.

Defenders of the market-oriented model, however, contend that commodification drives efficiency, innovation, and responsiveness to consumer demands. They argue that the competition inherent in a market-based system encourages providers to improve quality, reduce waste, and adapt to changing needs. Without the profit motive, they assert, the pace of medical advancements would slow, and the system would lack the dynamism necessary to meet the challenges of an aging population, emerging diseases, and technological change.

The commodification of healthcare reflects a broader ideological debate about the role of markets in addressing fundamental human needs. In the U.S., where capitalism shapes every facet of life, it is perhaps unsurprising that healthcare has become a market commodity. Yet this commodification is not without consequences. It shapes who receives care, how that care is delivered, and what priorities guide the system as a whole. As the debate over healthcare reform continues, the question remains: can a system built on market principles reconcile its profit motives with its obligation to serve the public good? Or will the commodification of healthcare deepen the divide between those who benefit from the system and those who are left behind?

Part 2: A System of Winners and Losers

Chapter 4: The Business of Medicine – Who Profits, Who Pays

Insurers occupy a central role in the American healthcare system, functioning as the primary gatekeepers of access to medical care. Their influence extends far beyond merely administering coverage; they shape the very framework within which patients, providers, and healthcare institutions operate. Insurance companies determine what treatments are covered, which providers are considered "in-network," and what portion of the costs will ultimately fall on patients. This power to mediate access to care situates insurers at the nexus of decision-making in the healthcare landscape, often leaving patients and providers constrained by their policies.

The health insurance market in the United States is characterized by a for-profit model that incentivizes cost containment and profit generation over comprehensive patient care. Insurers achieve profitability by carefully managing risk pools, setting premiums, and negotiating reimbursement rates with providers. These financial imperatives often lead to practices that prioritize the bottom line over accessibility. For example, insurers frequently employ utilization management techniques, such as requiring prior authorizations for treatments or imposing coverage limitations, which can delay or deny care. While such measures are justified as efforts to reduce waste and overuse of medical services, they often result in patients being denied timely, essential interventions.

For many Americans, access to health insurance is intricately tied to employment, creating a system where coverage is neither universal nor guaranteed. Employer-sponsored insurance remains the dominant source of coverage, but this linkage creates vulnerabilities. Losing a job often means losing health insurance, leaving millions uninsured or underinsured. Even those with insurance face high deductibles, copayments, and other out-of-pocket expenses that render care financially inaccessible. These financial barriers lead to a paradox: people with coverage may still forgo necessary treatments due to cost concerns, while the uninsured face even graver consequences, often delaying care until conditions worsen, leading to higher overall costs and poorer outcomes.

The insurance industry also plays a significant role in determining the structure and efficiency of healthcare delivery. By negotiating reimbursement rates with providers, insurers effectively dictate the economic viability of certain specialties, procedures, and services. Providers in lower-paying specialties or geographic regions with less favorable contracts are often left struggling to sustain their practices. Moreover, insurers' emphasis on cost control has fueled the rise of narrow networks, wherein patients are limited to a restricted list of in-network providers. While this approach is designed to reduce costs, it also limits patient choice and creates logistical hurdles for those seeking specialized or out-of-network care.

The administrative complexity imposed by the insurance system further compounds its gatekeeping role. Providers must navigate an intricate web of billing codes, claims processes, and reimbursement policies, diverting valuable time and resources away from patient care. The administrative burden of dealing with insurers contributes to burnout among healthcare professionals and inflates overall system costs. Studies consistently show that the United States spends more on healthcare administration than any other country, a disparity largely attributable to the complexities of private insurance.

Insurers have also played a pivotal role in the broader policy landscape, influencing the direction of healthcare reform. Their lobbying efforts have shaped legislation, including the Affordable Care Act (ACA), in ways that protect their interests. For instance, the ACA's individual mandate, which required most Americans to have health insurance, ensured a steady influx of customers into the market. While the ACA expanded coverage and implemented consumer protections, such as prohibiting discrimination based on pre-existing conditions, it also reinforced the centrality of private insurers in the system. Efforts to move toward single-payer or public option models have faced staunch opposition from the insurance industry, which stands to lose market share and profits under such reforms.

Insurers often defend their practices by pointing to their role in mitigating the rising costs of care. They argue that their cost-containment strategies are necessary to manage limited resources in a system plagued by inefficiencies and waste. By pooling risk and negotiating prices, insurers claim to provide a buffer against the exorbitant costs of care that would otherwise fall entirely on patients. However, this defense is tempered by the reality that insurers themselves contribute to these costs through high administrative overhead, marketing expenditures, and profit margins.

The relationship between insurers and other stakeholders in the healthcare system is both collaborative and contentious. While insurers negotiate with providers and pharmaceutical companies to lower costs, they also contribute to a fragmented system where pricing and decision-making lack transparency. Patients often find themselves caught in the crossfire, facing surprise bills or denied claims due to misaligned incentives between insurers and providers. This dynamic underscores the challenges of relying on private insurers as gatekeepers in a system ostensibly designed to prioritize health outcomes.

Despite their flaws, insurers remain an indispensable component of the current system, and any effort to reform healthcare must grapple with their entrenched role. Proposals to expand public options or transition to single-payer systems must address the significant disruption such changes would bring to the insurance industry. Similarly, efforts to regulate insurers more stringently, such as by capping premiums or requiring greater price transparency, must contend with the industry's political influence and economic power.

Insurers' position as gatekeepers of access reflects both the strengths and weaknesses of the American healthcare system. While they provide a mechanism for spreading risk and managing costs, their profit-driven model often prioritizes financial performance over equitable access to care. Patients, providers, and policymakers must navigate a system where the interests of insurers frequently shape outcomes. As debates about healthcare reform continue, the role of insurers will remain a focal point, emblematic of the broader tension between profit and patient-centered care in the business of medicine.

Pharmaceutical Companies – The Cost of Innovation

Pharmaceutical companies occupy a dual-edged role in the American healthcare system, representing both remarkable advancements in medical innovation and a persistent source of controversy due to high drug prices and opaque business practices. Positioned as the architects of modern medicine, these companies have delivered life-saving therapies, extended life expectancy, and transformed once-fatal diseases into manageable conditions. Yet, their profit-driven model often clashes with the public's need for affordable and equitable access to essential medications, illustrating the inherent tensions of a healthcare system rooted in capitalism.

The pharmaceutical industry's primary justification for high drug prices lies in the cost of innovation. Developing a new medication is an extraordinarily expensive and lengthy process, often spanning over a decade and costing billions of dollars. Research and development (R&D) expenses include early-stage discovery, preclinical testing, and extensive clinical trials to meet stringent regulatory requirements. For every successful drug brought to market, countless other compounds fail during testing, with no return on the substantial investments made. Pharmaceutical companies argue that high prices are necessary to recoup these costs and fund future innovations, maintaining the pipeline of breakthrough therapies that advance modern medicine.

However, the industry's pricing practices extend beyond covering R&D costs, revealing a profit-maximization strategy that prioritizes shareholder returns. The United States stands as an anomaly among developed nations, as it permits pharmaceutical companies to set drug prices with minimal government regulation. This freedom has resulted in some of the highest medication costs in the world, with patients often bearing the brunt of these expenses through out-of-pocket payments, high insurance premiums, or limited access to essential drugs. Critics argue that the industry's pricing practices disproportionately burden vulnerable populations, particularly the uninsured, those with chronic conditions, and low-income families.

One of the most contentious aspects of pharmaceutical pricing is the use of market exclusivity granted by patents. Patents, typically lasting 20 years from the date of filing, provide companies with a temporary monopoly on their products, allowing them to set prices without competition. While this exclusivity is intended to incentivize innovation, companies often exploit legal loopholes to extend their monopolies, a practice known as "evergreening." By making minor modifications to existing drugs or obtaining secondary patents for new uses, dosages, or delivery methods, pharmaceutical companies can prolong their control over lucrative markets, delaying the entry of more affordable generic alternatives.

The dynamics of pricing and exclusivity are further complicated by the role of middlemen, such as pharmacy benefit managers (PBMs), in the pharmaceutical supply chain. PBMs negotiate drug prices with manufacturers on behalf of insurers and employers, ostensibly to secure discounts and rebates. However, the opaque nature of these negotiations often obscures whether savings are passed on to patients or absorbed as profits by PBMs and insurers. This lack of transparency contributes to a fragmented system in which patients face rising costs without a clear understanding of the factors driving these increases.

In addition to pricing controversies, the industry has faced scrutiny over its marketing and promotional practices. Pharmaceutical companies spend billions annually on direct-to-consumer advertising and physician-targeted promotions, including sponsored research, speaking engagements, and free samples. While these strategies are intended to educate healthcare providers and patients about new treatments, they have been criticized for promoting overprescription and creating conflicts of interest. The opioid crisis, driven in part by aggressive marketing of pain medications, serves as a stark example of the devastating consequences that can arise when profit motives override public health considerations.

Despite these challenges, the pharmaceutical industry remains indispensable to the healthcare system, delivering innovations that save lives and improve quality of life. The rapid development of COVID-19 vaccines during the global pandemic showcased the industry's capacity for collaboration, speed, and scientific ingenuity. Partnerships between pharmaceutical companies, governments, and academic institutions enabled unprecedented progress, demonstrating that the profit motive can align with public health needs under the right circumstances. Yet, the pandemic also highlighted disparities in access to medications, as wealthier nations secured the majority of vaccine supplies while poorer countries faced shortages, underscoring the global inequities perpetuated by a market-driven system.

Efforts to address the high cost of medications have sparked ongoing debates about the role of government regulation and market intervention. Proposals such as allowing Medicare to negotiate drug prices, capping out-of-pocket costs for patients, and increasing transparency in pricing have garnered widespread support but face significant opposition from the pharmaceutical industry. The industry's lobbying efforts are among the most well-funded in the United States, with billions spent annually to influence legislation and protect its interests. This political power complicates reform efforts, as policymakers must navigate the competing pressures of public demand for affordability and the industry's warnings about the potential impact on innovation.

International comparisons offer valuable insights into alternative approaches to balancing innovation and affordability. Countries with centralized healthcare systems, such as the United Kingdom and Canada, employ price negotiation and cost-effectiveness analyses to ensure that medications are both accessible and financially sustainable. These models demonstrate that it is possible to incentivize innovation while maintaining accountability in pricing. However, importing such practices into the United States is challenging due to its decentralized, market-oriented system and the political influence of industry stakeholders.

The pharmaceutical industry's role in the American healthcare system exemplifies the broader tension between profit-driven innovation and equitable access to care. While the industry has achieved extraordinary scientific advancements, its pricing practices and business strategies often undermine the public's trust and exacerbate inequalities. Addressing these issues requires a nuanced approach that preserves the incentives for innovation while ensuring that life-saving medications are accessible to all who need them. Achieving this balance is a formidable task, but it is essential for creating a healthcare system that works not only for pharmaceutical companies but also for the patients they serve.

Hospitals – The Hub of Care Delivery

Hospitals represent the cornerstone of healthcare delivery, embodying both the promise and paradox of the American healthcare system. They are where life begins, ends, and is often saved. Yet, they are also institutions where care can come at an exorbitant financial cost, reflecting the complexities and contradictions of a profit-driven model. As hubs of advanced medical technology, specialized care, and community health services, hospitals sit at the nexus of healthcare's humanistic ideals and its economic realities.

The American hospital system is unique in its diverse ownership structures, encompassing public, private non-profit, and for-profit entities. Non-profit hospitals, which make up the majority, operate under the premise of reinvesting profits into the institution to improve care and serve the community. In contrast, for-profit hospitals prioritize shareholder returns, often focusing on lucrative services like elective surgeries or specialty care. Public hospitals, funded and operated by local or state governments, primarily serve low-income and uninsured populations. These distinctions create significant variability in access, quality, and financial practices across the hospital landscape.

At the heart of hospital operations lies a delicate balance between delivering high-quality care and maintaining financial viability. Hospitals are capital-intensive institutions, requiring substantial investments in infrastructure, technology, and staffing. The cost of maintaining state-of-the-art facilities and acquiring advanced medical equipment often drives hospitals to prioritize services that generate higher revenues. This economic imperative can result in the underprovision of less profitable services, such as mental health care or emergency treatment, despite their critical importance to community health.

The financial pressures faced by hospitals are exacerbated by the complexities of the American reimbursement system. Unlike many other developed nations with centralized healthcare financing, the U.S. relies on a fragmented mix of public and private payers. Medicare and Medicaid reimburse hospitals at rates often lower than the actual cost of providing care, compelling hospitals to negotiate higher payments from private insurers. This cost-shifting dynamic creates wide disparities in pricing, with uninsured patients frequently charged exorbitant rates as hospitals attempt to recover uncompensated care costs. The result is a pricing structure that is opaque, inconsistent, and often financially devastating for patients.

One of the most striking aspects of hospital economics is the phenomenon of "chargemasters"—internal pricing lists that dictate the initial cost of medical services. These prices, which often bear little resemblance to the actual costs of care, are used as starting points in negotiations with insurers. While most insured patients benefit from discounted rates through their coverage, uninsured individuals are typically billed the full chargemaster price, leading to shocking medical bills that can drive families into bankruptcy. Efforts to increase transparency, such as federal requirements for hospitals to publish their chargemasters, have revealed the staggering variability in prices between institutions but have done little to curb excessive billing practices.

The emphasis on profitability has also influenced hospital consolidation trends, with smaller hospitals merging into larger health systems or being acquired by corporate entities. Proponents of consolidation argue that it improves efficiency, reduces costs, and enhances care coordination. However, evidence suggests that consolidation often leads to reduced competition, higher prices, and diminished accountability. Patients in regions dominated by a single health system may face fewer choices, longer wait times, and limited bargaining power, underscoring the potential downsides of a highly concentrated hospital market.

Amid these financial and operational challenges, hospitals remain indispensable as centers of specialized care and innovation. They are where cutting-edge treatments are developed and delivered, from groundbreaking surgeries to experimental therapies. Academic medical centers, which combine clinical care, education, and research, play a pivotal role in advancing medical science and training the next generation of healthcare professionals. Yet, these institutions also grapple with the competing demands of academic rigor and financial sustainability, often relying on government funding, philanthropic contributions, and profitable service lines to support their missions.

Hospitals are also critical safety nets for vulnerable populations, particularly during public health crises. The COVID-19 pandemic underscored the indispensable role of hospitals as frontline responders, shouldering the burden of testing, treatment, and vaccination on an unprecedented scale. However, the pandemic also revealed systemic vulnerabilities, including staffing shortages, resource disparities, and financial instability. Many hospitals, especially rural and community-based institutions, faced closure or significant cutbacks due to pandemic-related revenue losses, exacerbating healthcare access issues in underserved areas.

The human element of hospital care is equally complex, as hospitals serve as workplaces for a diverse and highly skilled workforce. Nurses, physicians, technicians, and support staff operate under immense pressure, balancing the emotional and physical demands of patient care with systemic inefficiencies and administrative burdens. Burnout among healthcare workers has reached alarming levels, driven by long hours, inadequate staffing, and the strain of navigating bureaucratic hurdles. The well-being of hospital staff is inextricably linked to patient outcomes, highlighting the need for systemic reforms that prioritize both caregiver and patient needs.

Efforts to address the challenges facing hospitals have ranged from policy interventions to innovative care models. Value-based payment systems, which reward hospitals for quality and efficiency rather than volume of services, aim to realign financial incentives with patient outcomes. Community health initiatives, such as partnerships between hospitals and local organizations, seek to address social determinants of health and reduce reliance on costly emergency care. Technology also holds promise, with telemedicine, electronic health records, and data analytics offering new tools for improving care coordination and efficiency.

Despite these advancements, the American hospital system remains a microcosm of the broader tensions in U.S. healthcare. Hospitals exemplify the potential of medical science and the dedication of healthcare professionals, yet they are also sites of profound inequities and systemic inefficiencies. Reforming the hospital sector requires navigating these dual realities, ensuring that financial sustainability does not come at the expense of equitable access and high-quality care. Only by addressing these challenges can hospitals fulfill their role as the true hubs of care delivery, serving both the ideals of medicine and the needs of the communities they exist to support.

Providers – Caught in the Crossfire

At the heart of the healthcare system are its providers—physicians, nurses, therapists, and other professionals who deliver care directly to patients. They are the human touch in an industry increasingly dominated by corporate interests, complex regulations, and financial constraints. Providers represent the bridge between medical science and patient care, embodying the trust and empathy that define the therapeutic relationship. Yet, their role has become fraught with challenges that reflect the broader dysfunctions of the American healthcare system.

For providers, the practice of medicine is both a calling and a battleground. They enter the field motivated by a desire to heal, often enduring years of rigorous education and training to gain the expertise necessary to care for patients. However, once in the workforce, they find themselves navigating a labyrinth of administrative burdens, economic pressures, and ethical dilemmas. The day-to-day realities of modern healthcare often place them in the uncomfortable position of reconciling their professional values with the systemic constraints imposed by payers, hospitals, and government regulations.

One of the most significant pressures providers face is the increasing dominance of bureaucratic oversight in clinical practice. Electronic health records (EHRs), initially heralded as tools for improving efficiency and patient outcomes, have instead become symbols of provider burnout. Physicians spend hours documenting visits and fulfilling regulatory requirements, often at the expense of direct patient care. Studies have shown that for every hour providers spend with patients, they spend nearly two hours on administrative tasks, a ratio that undermines the therapeutic relationship and contributes to dissatisfaction and fatigue.

Providers also contend with the financial implications of healthcare delivery, which frequently require them to navigate the competing interests of insurers, hospitals, and patients. Insurers dictate the scope of covered services and reimbursement rates, compelling providers to justify treatments through extensive documentation and appeals. Simultaneously, hospitals and health systems impose productivity quotas and revenue targets, pressuring providers to see more patients in less time. This dynamic often forces providers into moral quandaries, where the quality of care they wish to deliver is constrained by the economic realities of the system.

The financial model of fee-for-service reimbursement, which incentivizes volume over value, further complicates the provider's role. While this system encourages the delivery of billable services, it often prioritizes procedures and interventions over preventive care and holistic treatment. Providers working under these conditions may feel torn between meeting productivity expectations and delivering patient-centered care. In response, some have embraced value-based care models that reward outcomes and efficiency, though these initiatives require significant investments in infrastructure and coordination that are not universally accessible.

Burnout among providers has emerged as a crisis within the healthcare workforce, with consequences that ripple across the system. Long hours, emotional labor, and the relentless pace of patient care take a toll on physical and mental health, leading to high rates of depression, anxiety, and even suicide among healthcare professionals. Burnout not only impacts providers' well-being but also compromises patient safety and care quality. Providers experiencing exhaustion and disengagement are more likely to make errors, struggle with communication, and leave the profession prematurely, exacerbating workforce shortages.

The financial realities of medical education compound these challenges, particularly for physicians. The cost of attending medical school in the United States often exceeds $200,000, leaving graduates with substantial debt. This financial burden influences career choices, driving many providers toward higher-paying specialties rather than primary care or underserved areas. The maldistribution of providers perpetuates disparities in access to care, as rural and low-income communities struggle to attract and retain healthcare professionals.

Despite these systemic pressures, providers remain committed to their patients, often going to extraordinary lengths to advocate for their needs. They are the ones who fight with insurers over denied claims, counsel patients through difficult diagnoses, and provide care in under-resourced settings. The resilience of providers is a testament to their dedication, yet it also underscores the unsustainable demands placed on them by a system that too often undervalues their contributions.

Efforts to address these challenges have gained momentum, driven by recognition of the critical role providers play in achieving a functional healthcare system. Policymakers and health systems have explored initiatives to reduce administrative burdens, such as streamlining prior authorization processes and redesigning EHR interfaces to prioritize usability. Programs aimed at combating burnout, including wellness initiatives, mental health support, and workload adjustments, have begun to address the human costs of care delivery.

Moreover, alternative payment models that align incentives with patient outcomes rather than service volume offer promise for reshaping the provider experience. These models, including Accountable Care Organizations (ACOs) and bundled payments, encourage care coordination and reduce unnecessary interventions. However, their success depends on robust infrastructure, interdisciplinary collaboration, and equitable implementation across diverse healthcare settings.

Providers also find hope in emerging technologies that enhance their ability to deliver care without adding to their workload. Artificial intelligence and machine learning tools hold potential for automating routine tasks, analyzing complex data, and supporting clinical decision-making. Telemedicine, accelerated by the COVID-19 pandemic, has expanded access to care while offering providers more flexibility in how they practice.

Ultimately, the future of healthcare depends on empowering providers to fulfill their role as caregivers, advocates, and innovators. This requires systemic reforms that address the root causes of provider dissatisfaction, from financial incentives to administrative complexity. It also demands a cultural shift within healthcare organizations, where provider well-being is prioritized alongside patient outcomes.

Providers stand at the intersection of policy, practice, and patient care, uniquely positioned to drive change from within the system. By supporting their resilience and amplifying their voices, the healthcare industry can create an environment where providers are not just surviving but thriving. In doing so, it can uphold the promise of medicine as a profession rooted in compassion, expertise, and the unwavering commitment to healing.

THE ROLE OF CORPORATE POWER AND MONOPOLIES

Corporate power and monopolies have deeply shaped the modern healthcare landscape, steering its priorities and outcomes in ways that often conflict with the principles of equitable care and accessibility. Over the decades, the consolidation of power among a handful of dominant players—whether insurers, pharmaceutical companies, or hospital systems—has created a structure that prioritizes profit margins over patient welfare. This concentration of influence has far-reaching implications, dictating not only the cost and availability of care but also the innovation, quality, and ethical underpinnings of the system.

The rise of monopolistic tendencies in healthcare is perhaps most evident in the pharmaceutical sector, where a few multinational corporations control the production and distribution of essential drugs. These companies leverage patent protections and market exclusivity to maintain high prices, arguing that such strategies are necessary to recoup the vast investments required for research and development. While it is true that the discovery and approval of new treatments involve significant costs, the balance between profit and accessibility often skews disproportionately toward the former. For instance, life-saving medications like insulin remain prohibitively expensive for many patients in the United States, despite being relatively inexpensive to produce. Such pricing practices highlight the tension between innovation and exploitation, where monopolistic control can hinder equitable access to essential therapies.

The hospital sector has similarly seen an alarming trend toward consolidation, with smaller, independent facilities being absorbed into larger health systems. These mergers are frequently justified as a means of achieving economies of scale, improving care coordination, and increasing operational efficiency. However, studies have shown that consolidation often leads to higher prices for patients and payers without corresponding improvements in care quality. Large hospital networks wield significant bargaining power in negotiations with insurers, enabling them to set higher reimbursement rates. This dynamic contributes to the overall escalation of healthcare costs, creating financial barriers for patients and straining public and private insurance programs.

Insurers, too, have leveraged their position to consolidate influence, creating regional or national monopolies that limit competition and choice. In many areas, a single insurer dominates the market, effectively dictating the terms of coverage and reimbursement. This lack of competition stifles innovation and leaves consumers with few alternatives, often forcing them to accept higher premiums, narrower networks, and restrictive policies. While insurers claim to act as stewards of cost control by negotiating with providers and pharmaceutical companies, their profit-driven motives frequently align more closely with shareholder interests than with patient care.

Corporate power also manifests in the vertical integration of healthcare entities, where organizations expand their reach across multiple facets of the industry. For example, insurers acquiring pharmacy benefit managers (PBMs) or hospital systems opening their own insurance plans blur traditional boundaries, creating complex conglomerates that control both the provision and financing of care. While such integration promises streamlined services and reduced inefficiencies, it often results in opaque pricing structures, conflicts of interest, and reduced accountability.

Monopolistic practices extend beyond pricing and market dominance to influence policymaking and regulation. Through extensive lobbying efforts, corporate entities shape legislation to protect their interests, often at the expense of systemic reform. The pharmaceutical industry, for instance, has spent billions lobbying Congress to block measures like drug price negotiation or importation of cheaper medications from abroad. Similarly, hospital associations advocate against policies that would increase transparency in billing or expand competitive alternatives like publicly funded health options. This political influence underscores the entrenchment of corporate power in shaping the rules of the game, ensuring the preservation of their dominance within the system.

The consequences of this concentration of power are felt most acutely by patients and providers, who navigate a system designed to prioritize profits over care. Patients bear the financial burden of inflated prices and limited options, often delaying or forgoing treatment due to cost. Providers, on the other hand, grapple with the constraints imposed by corporate interests, from restrictive formularies dictated by PBMs to productivity quotas set by hospital administrators. These pressures distort clinical decision-making, forcing compromises that erode trust and diminish the integrity of care.

Efforts to counteract monopolistic power and promote competition face significant challenges but are essential to rebalancing the system. Regulatory measures such as antitrust enforcement, price transparency laws, and policies to encourage generic drug competition represent critical steps in addressing these imbalances. For example, breaking up large hospital networks or restricting vertical integration could restore competition and empower smaller, community-focused entities to thrive. Similarly, reforms to patent laws and drug pricing mechanisms could ensure that innovation remains a priority without sacrificing accessibility.

In addition to regulatory action, fostering consumer and provider advocacy is crucial for challenging the dominance of corporate interests. Empowering patients with tools to compare prices, understand billing, and choose alternative care options can create demand-driven pressure for transparency and fairness. Providers, too, play a vital role in advocating for systemic change, leveraging their collective voice to push back against exploitative practices and prioritize patient welfare.

The unchecked power of monopolies and corporate interests poses a fundamental threat to the ideals of a fair and functional healthcare system. Addressing this imbalance requires a multifaceted approach that combines policy reforms, market restructuring, and cultural shifts within the industry. By challenging the status quo, it is possible to realign healthcare with its core mission: delivering accessible, affordable, and high-quality care to all.

CHAPTER 5: THE DISPARITIES OF CARE

In the United States, the healthcare system exists as a paradox: a marvel of modern medicine capable of extraordinary achievements, yet deeply divided by systemic inequities. To understand this duality, one must explore the lived experiences of those it serves—and fails. In a thriving urban suburb, a patient facing a cardiac emergency can expect immediate access to state-of-the-art facilities, a network of specialists, and cutting-edge interventions. Meanwhile, in a rural community or underserved city neighborhood, someone in a similar crisis may confront long travel distances to the nearest hospital, understaffed clinics, or outdated equipment. The disparity is not merely one of inconvenience but of life and death, with geography, income, and social status serving as the gatekeepers of health outcomes.

These two realities are neither accidents nor anomalies. They are the direct products of a system where healthcare has been shaped by market forces rather than principles of equity. The affluent enjoy access to comprehensive insurance plans, concierge care, and the latest medical technologies, reinforcing a cycle of privilege that keeps them healthier, longer. Conversely, millions of Americans in marginalized communities struggle to secure even basic services, hindered by a web of systemic barriers that reflect deeper societal inequalities.

The contrast is stark, but its roots run deep. From urban centers with gleaming hospitals to rural stretches marked by the closure of community facilities, the American healthcare system reflects the broader economic divides of the nation. It serves as a mirror of a society that rewards wealth with opportunity and consigns the less fortunate to lives of precarity. In this landscape, the outcomes of care are not determined solely by medical expertise or technological advancements but by the structural inequities that dictate who gets to access them.

Why does this system, so advanced in its capabilities, so often fail to meet its promise for vast swathes of the population? The answer lies not only in policy decisions but in the economic and political priorities that have historically treated healthcare as a commodity rather than a right. To delve into these dual realities is to confront a system where success and failure coexist, defined not by chance but by design.

Healthcare Deserts: Where Geography Determines Access

In the vast and varied geography of the United States, access to healthcare is not a universal guarantee but a privilege dictated by one's zip code. Healthcare deserts—regions with limited or nonexistent access to medical facilities—are stark reminders of this inequality. These areas, predominantly rural but also present in urban centers, are characterized by the absence of primary care providers, specialists, and hospitals, leaving residents with few options beyond overburdened clinics or distant healthcare facilities.

In rural America, healthcare deserts stretch across vast expanses, where hospitals are few and far between, and the nearest doctor might be a county away. The closures of rural hospitals, a phenomenon accelerated in recent decades by financial insolvency and policy changes, have exacerbated this crisis.

These closures often occur in communities where populations are aging, incomes are lower, and a significant portion of residents rely on Medicare or Medicaid—programs that reimburse providers at lower rates, making their operation financially unsustainable. The result is a vicious cycle: as facilities shut their doors, populations are left with reduced access, leading to worse health outcomes and, in turn, diminishing the economic viability of these communities further.

Urban healthcare deserts present a different but equally concerning reality. In cities, the lack of healthcare access is not due to geographic isolation but systemic neglect of impoverished neighborhoods. Safety-net hospitals, often located in these areas, are overwhelmed by demand and underfunded, struggling to provide care for uninsured or underinsured populations. Pharmacies are scarce in these regions, leading to "pharmacy deserts" where even basic medications become difficult to obtain. Public transportation systems, designed with little consideration for healthcare access, further isolate residents from the care they need.

The consequences of healthcare deserts are dire. Preventative care is often inaccessible, leading to advanced stages of illness by the time medical attention is sought. Chronic conditions like diabetes and hypertension go unmanaged, mental health needs remain unmet, and maternal mortality rates rise in areas where obstetric services are no longer available. These outcomes are not evenly distributed but disproportionately affect low-income individuals and communities of color, compounding existing health disparities.

The existence of healthcare deserts reveals the spatial dimensions of inequality in the U.S. healthcare system. While some regions benefit from an abundance of providers and resources, others languish in neglect, creating a chasm in health outcomes that mirrors the broader socioeconomic divides of the nation. Geography, in this context, is not merely a backdrop but a determining factor in who lives, who suffers, and who dies.

Racial Inequalities in Healthcare

Racial inequalities in healthcare are deeply entrenched in the fabric of the American healthcare system, reflecting a legacy of structural racism, historical neglect, and ongoing systemic barriers. These disparities manifest across every dimension of care, from access to treatment outcomes, and are as pervasive as they are devastating. While the principles of medicine emphasize equality and justice, the lived experiences of many racial and ethnic minorities tell a different story—one of exclusion, mistrust, and inequity.

The roots of racial disparities in healthcare trace back to the history of segregation and discrimination in American society. From the exclusion of Black patients from white-only hospitals during the Jim Crow era to the unethical medical experiments such as the Tuskegee Syphilis Study, the healthcare system has long marginalized communities of color. This historical context shapes contemporary healthcare practices and attitudes, fueling a persistent mistrust of medical institutions among many minority populations.

The inequalities are particularly stark when examining access to care. Black and Hispanic Americans are significantly more likely than their white counterparts to be uninsured, limiting their ability to afford preventative and routine medical services. Even for those with insurance, barriers such as a lack of culturally competent providers, language difficulties, and implicit bias in medical decision-making create additional hurdles. For Native American communities, who are guaranteed healthcare through treaties and federal obligations, chronic underfunding of the Indian Health Service leaves many without adequate resources, facilities, or specialists.

The disparities extend beyond access to the quality of care received. Minority patients frequently face implicit biases from healthcare providers, which can influence diagnosis, treatment decisions, and pain management. Studies consistently show that Black patients are less likely than white patients to receive appropriate treatments for conditions such as heart disease, cancer, and pain management. For example, the persistent myth that Black individuals have higher pain thresholds continues to result in inadequate pain relief for many Black patients, perpetuating cycles of suffering and mistrust.

These inequities are not solely the result of individual biases but are embedded in the system itself. Hospital closures and resource allocation disproportionately affect minority neighborhoods, compounding the challenges of healthcare access. Health outcomes such as maternal mortality highlight these disparities with devastating clarity: Black women in the United States are three times more likely to die from pregnancy-related complications than white women, regardless of income or education level.

The COVID-19 pandemic laid bare the systemic nature of these inequities, as communities of color experienced disproportionately high rates of infection, hospitalization, and death. Underlying health disparities—such as higher rates of diabetes, hypertension, and asthma—combined with social determinants of health like crowded housing, essential jobs, and limited access to testing and vaccines, created a perfect storm of vulnerability.

Efforts to address racial disparities in healthcare require more than incremental reforms; they demand systemic change. Cultural competency training, equitable resource distribution, and policy initiatives aimed at expanding coverage are critical steps. However, these efforts must also contend with the broader social determinants of health—education, housing, and employment opportunities—that perpetuate health disparities.

Racial inequalities in healthcare are not anomalies; they are the inevitable result of a system designed without equity at its core. Addressing these disparities requires confronting uncomfortable truths about the ways in which race and racism continue to shape health and healthcare in America. The question is not merely how to make the system fairer, but how to dismantle the barriers that have long prevented it from serving all equally.

THE PLIGHT OF THE UNINSURED

The plight of the uninsured is one of the most glaring and persistent failures of the American healthcare system. In a nation that boasts cutting-edge medical innovations and some of the most advanced treatment capabilities in the world, millions of people remain locked out of the system, unable to access even basic care. For these individuals, the absence of insurance is not merely an inconvenience; it is a profound determinant of their health outcomes, financial stability, and overall quality of life.

The uninsured are not a monolithic group but a diverse demographic comprising low-wage workers, part-time employees, small business owners, and the unemployed. Many earn too much to qualify for Medicaid yet too little to afford private insurance or to weather the high premiums of marketplace plans. For these individuals, falling through the cracks is not accidental—it is the inevitable result of a system that ties access to healthcare to employment, wealth, and state-level policies.

The consequences of being uninsured are devastating. Without access to preventive care, many are forced to forgo routine screenings, vaccinations, and early interventions that could prevent serious illnesses. Chronic conditions such as diabetes, hypertension, and asthma often remain unmanaged, leading to complications that are both debilitating and costly. When uninsured individuals do seek care, it is often in emergency rooms, the most expensive and least efficient setting, which shifts costs to hospitals and insured patients, further straining the system.

Financial ruin is another common outcome for the uninsured. A single medical emergency—an accident, an unexpected diagnosis, or a hospitalization—can spiral into a lifetime of debt. Medical bills are a leading cause of bankruptcy in the United States, and the uninsured bear the brunt of this burden. Unlike those with insurance, who benefit from negotiated rates, the uninsured are often charged the full sticker price for services, compounding the financial inequities they already face.

Geography further complicates the plight of the uninsured. States that chose not to expand Medicaid under the Affordable Care Act (ACA) are home to a disproportionate share of uninsured residents. In these states, adults without dependent children and those earning slightly above the federal poverty line remain excluded from coverage, creating a patchwork system where access to healthcare is determined by state borders rather than need. This disparity underscores the fragmented nature of American healthcare, where political ideology often outweighs public health priorities.

The uninsured population is also more likely to consist of racial and ethnic minorities, amplifying the inequities already present in the healthcare system. Immigrants, particularly undocumented individuals, face even greater hurdles, as they are excluded from Medicaid and most ACA provisions. For these groups, fear of deportation or discrimination often deters them from seeking care, even in emergencies, exacerbating health disparities.

The psychological toll of being uninsured cannot be overstated. The constant anxiety of knowing that an illness or injury could lead to financial catastrophe weighs heavily on individuals and families. Parents must make impossible choices between paying for a child's healthcare or meeting other basic needs like housing and food. This chronic stress, in turn, contributes to worse health outcomes, creating a vicious cycle of vulnerability.

Reforms such as the ACA have made significant strides in reducing the uninsured rate, yet gaps remain stubbornly persistent. Employer-sponsored insurance, the backbone of the American system, fails to reach those in unstable or low-paying jobs, while marketplace subsidies are often insufficient to make coverage affordable. Safety-net programs and free clinics attempt to fill the void, but their resources are limited, and their reach is inconsistent.

The uninsured represent the harshest critique of a system that prioritizes profit over people. Their plight exposes the fundamental inequities of a market-based healthcare model, where access is treated as a commodity rather than a right. Addressing their needs requires not only expanding coverage but also reimagining the very structure of American healthcare. Until that happens, the uninsured will remain emblematic of a system that works brilliantly for some and catastrophically for others.

THE INTERSECTION OF SOCIOECONOMIC STATUS AND HEALTH

Socioeconomic status (SES) is one of the most powerful determinants of health in the United States, shaping not only access to care but also the very conditions that influence whether individuals thrive or suffer. While health is often discussed in terms of individual choices and behaviors, the reality is that a person's income, education level, occupation, and social standing create the framework within which those choices are made. In the United States, where healthcare operates as a market commodity, the intersection of SES and health is especially stark, revealing a system that amplifies disparities rather than mitigating them.

Low-income individuals face a cascade of challenges that make maintaining good health exceedingly difficult. For many, the financial strain of meeting basic needs such as housing, food, and transportation takes precedence over preventive care or managing chronic conditions. These trade-offs mean that routine check-ups, dental visits, and prescription medications are often viewed as luxuries rather than necessities. Poor housing conditions—ranging from exposure to mold and pests to overcrowding—create environments ripe for respiratory illnesses and infectious diseases. Limited access to nutritious food, often compounded by the prevalence of "food deserts" in low-income neighborhoods, leads to diets high in processed and sugary foods, contributing to obesity, diabetes, and heart disease.

Employment further complicates the relationship between SES and health. Many low-wage jobs do not offer health insurance, paid sick leave, or flexible work schedules, leaving workers vulnerable to both financial strain and untreated health issues. When illness strikes, the lack of job security can mean choosing between a paycheck and personal well-being, perpetuating cycles of poor health and economic instability. Moreover, physically demanding jobs with high levels of stress, such as those in construction, agriculture, or service industries, often lead to injuries and long-term health problems, while offering little in the way of employer-supported care.

Education, a key component of SES, plays a pivotal role in determining health outcomes. Those with lower educational attainment are less likely to have the knowledge or resources to navigate the complexities of the healthcare system. They may struggle to understand medical instructions, adhere to treatment plans, or advocate for themselves in clinical settings. Furthermore, education is closely tied to income and employment opportunities, creating a reinforcing loop where limited education constrains access to the very factors that could improve health outcomes.

The disparities are not just material but systemic, with SES influencing how individuals are treated within the healthcare system itself. Studies consistently show that patients from lower socioeconomic backgrounds receive different levels of care compared to their wealthier counterparts, even when presenting with the same conditions. Implicit bias among healthcare providers, combined with structural barriers such as insurance status or ability to pay, results in delayed diagnoses, reduced access to specialists, and poorer overall outcomes for low-income patients. The phenomenon of "social triage," where providers may subconsciously prioritize patients perceived as having greater social value or resources, further deepens these inequities.

The consequences of the SES-health intersection extend beyond individual outcomes to the broader community. Neighborhoods with concentrated poverty often suffer from underfunded hospitals, clinics, and public health initiatives, creating healthcare deserts where access to even basic services is limited. The result is a vicious cycle in which poor health outcomes reinforce economic disadvantage, while economic disadvantage perpetuates poor health outcomes—a cycle that is both morally troubling and economically costly.

Socioeconomic disparities in health are not confined to any one racial or ethnic group, but they intersect with racial inequities in ways that magnify the challenges faced by marginalized communities. For example, Black, Latino, and Indigenous populations in the United States are disproportionately represented among low-income groups, making them more likely to experience the dual burdens of racial and socioeconomic inequities. This intersectionality compounds barriers to care, exacerbates mistrust in the healthcare system, and deepens the chasm between those who can access quality healthcare and those who cannot.

Efforts to address the intersection of SES and health must go beyond expanding insurance coverage or increasing the number of healthcare providers. They require a holistic approach that acknowledges and addresses the root causes of socioeconomic inequities. Policies that increase access to affordable housing, improve educational opportunities, and ensure living wages are as integral to improving health outcomes as reforms within the healthcare system itself. Programs that integrate healthcare with social services, providing patients with resources to address housing, food insecurity, and employment challenges, represent one of the most promising ways to break the cycle of poverty and poor health.

The intersection of SES and health in the United States underscores the limits of a market-driven system. While wealthier individuals can leverage their resources to access high-quality care, those at the bottom of the socioeconomic ladder face a fundamentally different reality—one marked by systemic neglect and limited opportunity. Addressing these disparities requires more than incremental change; it demands a reimagining of how health and well-being are valued in a society where economic status remains one of the most powerful predictors of life expectancy and quality of life.

STRUCTURAL DRIVERS OF DISPARITY: POLICIES AND PRACTICES

The structural drivers of healthcare disparity in the United States are deeply embedded in the policies, practices, and historical frameworks that govern the system. These drivers extend beyond individual behavior or localized inequities, reflecting a broader network of systemic issues that perpetuate inequality. Understanding these structural forces is crucial for addressing the root causes of disparities rather than merely treating their symptoms. Policies, institutional practices, and economic structures create an environment where healthcare inequities are not accidental but are instead the predictable outcomes of deliberate decisions.

One of the most significant structural drivers of disparity is the fragmented nature of the U.S. healthcare system. Unlike many industrialized nations with centralized, universal healthcare models, the American system is a patchwork of public and private programs, each with its own eligibility criteria, funding mechanisms, and service coverage. This fragmentation disproportionately affects marginalized populations, who often fall through the cracks of a system that was never designed to prioritize equitable access. For example, individuals earning just above the income threshold for Medicaid may lack the means to afford private insurance, leaving them effectively uninsured. Similarly, undocumented immigrants are excluded from most public programs, despite often being among the most vulnerable to poor health outcomes.

The design of employer-sponsored insurance has also played a central role in cementing disparities. This system, which ties access to healthcare to stable employment, inherently disadvantages those in part-time, low-wage, or precarious jobs. Workers in these positions are often from marginalized racial and socioeconomic groups, exacerbating their lack of access to care. Furthermore, industries dominated by these workers frequently offer limited or no benefits, creating structural barriers that are almost impossible for individuals to overcome without significant systemic reform.

Housing policy, often viewed as separate from healthcare, has profound implications for health disparities. Zoning laws, redlining practices, and urban renewal projects have historically segregated marginalized populations into neighborhoods with fewer healthcare resources, higher exposure to environmental hazards, and inadequate public health infrastructure. These structural inequities contribute to the phenomenon of "healthcare deserts," where entire communities lack access to primary care, specialty services, or even emergency medical facilities. The geography of healthcare access is thus a reflection of decades of policy decisions that prioritized economic development or racial segregation over equitable public health planning.

The role of federal and state legislation in shaping healthcare inequities cannot be overlooked. Policies such as the Affordable Care Act (ACA) have attempted to reduce disparities, yet their impact is uneven due to the decentralization of the system. For example, the ACA's Medicaid expansion aimed to increase access for low-income populations, but its implementation was left to individual states, resulting in a patchwork of coverage. States that chose not to expand Medicaid have left millions without access to affordable care, disproportionately affecting Black, Latino, and rural populations. This legislative inconsistency highlights how policy decisions at multiple levels of government perpetuate unequal healthcare access.

Economic incentives within the healthcare system further entrench disparities. The profit-driven model incentivizes providers to focus on high-revenue services, such as specialized surgeries or advanced diagnostics, often at the expense of primary and preventive care. This prioritization creates a resource imbalance, with well-funded hospitals and clinics clustered in affluent areas, while underfunded facilities struggle to meet basic needs in low-income and rural communities. Additionally, private insurance companies often design networks that exclude providers serving marginalized populations, leaving many patients with limited options for care.

Discriminatory practices, both overt and covert, within the healthcare system exacerbate these structural disparities. Implicit bias among healthcare providers can lead to unequal treatment, such as underdiagnosis of pain in Black patients or dismissive attitudes toward low-income individuals. These biases are not isolated incidents but are rooted in systemic issues, such as the lack of diversity in medical training and leadership, that perpetuate unequal care. Moreover, policies that link healthcare reimbursement to patient satisfaction scores may unintentionally disadvantage providers serving marginalized populations, as these metrics often fail to account for the systemic barriers their patients face.

The privatization of healthcare administration also plays a significant role in maintaining disparities. Private insurers, pharmaceutical companies, and hospital systems wield enormous influence over policy and resource allocation, often prioritizing profitability over equitable access. The lobbying power of these entities shapes legislative agendas, ensuring that reforms threatening their revenue streams are diluted or blocked entirely. For example, efforts to control prescription drug prices or mandate universal coverage have repeatedly faced staunch opposition from industry groups, leaving marginalized populations to bear the brunt of high costs and limited access.

Systemic underinvestment in public health infrastructure is a critical driver of disparity. Chronic underfunding of public health agencies, community health programs, and preventive care initiatives limits their ability to address the root causes of health inequities. This underinvestment is often a political decision, reflecting priorities that favor short-term cost savings over long-term health outcomes. For marginalized communities, this means fewer resources to combat chronic diseases, manage infectious outbreaks, or address social determinants of health.

Addressing the structural drivers of disparity requires a paradigm shift in how healthcare is conceptualized and delivered. Rather than focusing solely on individual behavior or market-based solutions, policymakers and stakeholders must confront the systemic inequities embedded in the system's design. This includes rethinking the role of profit in healthcare, investing in public health infrastructure, and implementing policies that prioritize equity over efficiency. Only by addressing these structural drivers can the United States begin to dismantle the disparities that have long defined its healthcare system.

HUMAN CONSEQUENCES: PERSONAL STORIES AND CASE STUDIES

The human consequences of systemic disparities in American healthcare are often obscured by statistics and policy debates. Yet behind every number lies a story, a lived experience that underscores the real toll of inequity. These personal accounts and case studies illuminate the profound impact of a system that consistently prioritizes profit and structural efficiency over equitable access to care. They remind us that disparities are not abstract concepts but daily realities with life-altering implications for millions of individuals and families.

Consider Maria, a middle-aged Latina woman living in a rural healthcare desert. Her closest hospital is over an hour away, and the local clinic, understaffed and underfunded, operates on a part-time schedule. Maria suffers from diabetes, a condition manageable with consistent medical care and access to insulin. However, the limited resources in her area and the high out-of-pocket cost of her medication make proper management impossible. She rationed her insulin to make it last, a dangerous but necessary decision, until one day she fell into a diabetic coma. Maria survived but lost her job due to prolonged absence during her recovery, plunging her family deeper into financial insecurity. Her story exemplifies the compounded vulnerabilities created by geographical isolation, economic hardship, and the structural failings of a fragmented healthcare system.

Then there's Darnell, a young Black man who avoids seeking medical attention even when he feels unwell. His distrust stems from a lifetime of dismissive encounters with healthcare providers, who often downplayed his symptoms or attributed them to his lifestyle without proper investigation. When Darnell was finally diagnosed with hypertension, it was only after an emergency room visit for chest pain. By then, the condition had progressed significantly, requiring costly and invasive interventions. Darnell's experience highlights how racial bias within the system discourages timely care, exacerbating conditions that might have been managed with earlier intervention.

In another case, the Hernandez family faces the insurmountable challenge of navigating the healthcare system as uninsured immigrants. Their son, Miguel, was born with a congenital heart defect requiring regular monitoring and potential surgical intervention. With no access to employer-sponsored insurance and ineligible for Medicaid, the family cobbles together funds for each appointment through community support and personal sacrifice. Despite their efforts, delays in care due to financial constraints lead to complications that might have been preventable with consistent treatment. Miguel's story showcases the plight of the uninsured, whose health outcomes are often determined more by financial status than medical need.

Healthcare disparities also extend to the very people delivering care. Jasmine, a nurse in an urban safety-net hospital, works long hours with limited resources to serve a predominantly low-income population. Burnout is common among her colleagues, who feel the weight of trying to meet overwhelming demand in an underfunded system. Jasmine often struggles with feelings of guilt and helplessness when she cannot provide the level of care she knows her patients deserve. Her story underscores the hidden toll disparities take on healthcare workers, who must navigate systemic inadequacies alongside their patients.

These personal narratives intersect with broader systemic issues, such as the high cost of care and the prioritization of market-driven solutions over human-centered policies. For instance, the case of Brian Thompson, a middle-class father diagnosed with cancer, illustrates how even those who seemingly "play by the rules" can fall victim to financial ruin. Despite having employer-sponsored insurance, the out-of-pocket costs for his treatments and medications quickly depleted the family's savings. Forced to choose between paying for care and covering basic living expenses, Brian's story is a stark reminder that healthcare disparities are not limited to the uninsured or the marginalized—they permeate every layer of society.

The consequences of these inequities ripple outward, affecting not only individuals but entire communities. In neighborhoods plagued by healthcare deserts, preventable conditions such as hypertension, diabetes, and asthma become endemic, perpetuating cycles of poor health and economic instability. These disparities contribute to intergenerational health inequities, where children born into underserved communities face higher risks of chronic illness and reduced life expectancy.

Personal stories like these reveal the urgent need for systemic change. They highlight how the structural flaws of the U.S. healthcare system translate into lived realities, marked by pain, loss, and unmet potential. More importantly, they serve as a call to action, demanding that policymakers, healthcare providers, and society as a whole confront the human cost of inaction. By centering these stories in the discourse on healthcare reform, we can shift the conversation from abstract policy debates to the tangible lives at stake, fostering a deeper understanding of what is truly at risk.

WHY THE SYSTEM WORKS WELL FOR SOME

The U.S. healthcare system, despite its glaring inequities, functions exceptionally well for certain segments of the population, reflecting its design as a market-driven enterprise rather than a universal right. For those with access to robust insurance coverage, financial resources, and proximity to high-quality facilities, the system offers unparalleled levels of care. This reality highlights the dual nature of American healthcare: it can be both world-class and deeply exclusionary, depending on one's position within its economic and social hierarchies.

For affluent individuals, the healthcare system provides near-instant access to state-of-the-art treatments and cutting-edge technologies. Private insurance plans, often provided as part of lucrative employment packages, allow patients to choose their physicians and facilities, bypass long wait times, and receive personalized care. The concierge medicine model takes this a step further, offering elite patients exclusive 24/7 access to primary care providers, detailed wellness plans, and even direct coordination of specialist appointments. These services, tailored to the individual, exemplify the system's capacity to deliver optimal outcomes when resources are not a limiting factor.

Take, for example, the case of a Silicon Valley executive diagnosed with an early-stage but aggressive form of cancer. Armed with premium insurance and considerable personal wealth, he could immediately consult with top oncologists across the country, access experimental therapies, and undergo treatments in facilities equipped with the latest technology. His care team worked in seamless coordination, focusing entirely on his recovery without the delays or compromises that plague less-privileged patients. The outcome: remission within a year, achieved through resources unattainable for the vast majority.

The system also rewards those with employer-sponsored insurance, particularly those in industries offering comprehensive benefits packages. Employees in such roles can access preventive care, routine screenings, and specialist visits with relative ease. This advantage not only improves immediate health outcomes but also fosters long-term wellness by catching and addressing conditions early. The tax incentives offered to employers for providing such benefits further solidify this dynamic, perpetuating a tiered system where health is closely tied to employment type and status.

Geography plays an equally significant role in determining for whom the system works. Urban centers, particularly those with academic medical institutions, serve as hubs for cutting-edge research and high-quality care. Residents in these areas benefit from proximity to specialized facilities and a concentration of skilled providers. For example, cities like Boston, Houston, and New York are home to world-renowned hospitals that attract patients from across the globe. Those fortunate enough to live nearby enjoy access to treatments that set global standards for excellence.

The pharmaceutical industry's vast resources and innovation pipeline further amplify the benefits available to the system's winners. For patients with excellent insurance or the means to pay out-of-pocket, breakthrough medications and therapies offer life-saving solutions that were unimaginable a few decades ago. The rapid development of mRNA vaccines during the COVID-19 pandemic demonstrated how the U.S. healthcare system, fueled by significant private and public investment, could respond with unprecedented speed and efficacy. However, the accessibility of such advancements remains uneven, with cost serving as the primary gatekeeper.

Even within the broader population, certain groups derive significant benefits from government programs like Medicare and Medicaid. While these programs are often criticized for their limitations, they provide essential coverage for millions of elderly, disabled, and low-income Americans. For seniors, Medicare represents a critical lifeline, enabling access to routine and specialized care that would otherwise be financially prohibitive. However, the disparities even within these programs reflect broader systemic inequities, as the level of care often hinges on supplemental coverage or state-specific Medicaid policies.

The system's functionality for these privileged groups underscores its inherent design: a model that prioritizes innovation, efficiency, and outcomes for those who can afford to participate fully. Yet this success comes at a cost. The same market mechanisms that drive excellence for some simultaneously exclude or marginalize others. The resources channeled into concierge medicine, high-tech facilities, and groundbreaking therapies for a select few often divert attention and funding from broader systemic reforms that could benefit the entire population.

Moreover, the system's reliance on profit motives ensures that those who can pay the most will always receive the best care, reinforcing cycles of inequality. This dynamic is not incidental but rather intrinsic to the market-oriented framework of American healthcare. The beneficiaries of the system are, in effect, subsidized by its failures, as the costs of uncompensated care for the uninsured or underinsured are absorbed through higher premiums and service charges.

For those who thrive under the current system, it is easy to overlook the structural inequities that sustain it. The efficiency, quality, and innovation experienced by the fortunate few are a stark contrast to the systemic neglect faced by the uninsured, the marginalized, and those trapped in healthcare deserts. This bifurcation is not a bug but a feature—a testament to a system that works exceptionally well for some while leaving many others behind. Understanding this duality is essential to any discussion of reform, as it reveals both the system's potential and its profound limitations.

Ethical and Practical Implications of Inequality

The ethical and practical implications of inequality in the U.S. healthcare system are profound, challenging the nation's moral compass while undermining its broader economic and social stability. At the heart of the issue lies a fundamental question: to what extent should a person's health and well-being be contingent on their socioeconomic status, race, or geographic location? The system's inequities not only raise pressing moral concerns but also create practical inefficiencies that ripple across society, affecting everyone—whether directly or indirectly.

From an ethical standpoint, the disparities within the healthcare system starkly contrast with core values often espoused in American society: equality, fairness, and the right to life, liberty, and the pursuit of happiness. Healthcare, arguably central to these ideals, remains inaccessible for many due to systemic barriers. This inequity highlights a troubling reality: in a profit-driven healthcare model, the value of a life often correlates with an individual's economic productivity or ability to pay. The prioritization of profits over patients perpetuates a system where access to care is treated as a privilege rather than a right, leading to preventable suffering and death among the marginalized.

The uninsured and underinsured bear the brunt of this inequality, facing impossible choices between seeking necessary medical attention and avoiding financial ruin. For these individuals, the system's failings are not abstract but visceral, manifesting in skipped treatments, unmanaged chronic illnesses, and premature mortality. The ethical dilemma becomes even more acute when considering the racial and socioeconomic dimensions of these disparities.

Communities of color and low-income populations disproportionately experience these systemic failures, a legacy of historical discrimination and structural racism that persists in modern policy and practice.

The ethical implications extend beyond individual experiences to the broader societal message these inequalities convey. When millions lack access to basic care while others enjoy the benefits of a system catering to their every need, it reinforces a hierarchy of human worth. The social fabric frays as trust in institutions erodes, fostering cynicism, resentment, and division. The healthcare system, intended to heal, instead becomes a mirror reflecting deeper societal inequities.

Beyond the moral considerations, the practical consequences of inequality in healthcare are equally dire. A system that excludes large swathes of the population from adequate care is inherently inefficient and unsustainable. Delayed or forgone treatments often result in more severe health issues down the line, requiring expensive emergency interventions that could have been avoided through preventive care. These costs are absorbed by the system through higher insurance premiums, increased government spending on uncompensated care, and diminished economic productivity due to a sicker workforce. In this way, the consequences of inequality ripple outward, affecting even those who appear to benefit most from the current system.

Public health crises further expose the fragility of a system built on inequality. The COVID-19 pandemic, for example, starkly illustrated how gaps in healthcare access can amplify the spread of disease and deepen its impact. Communities with limited access to care experienced higher infection rates, worse outcomes, and slower recovery, exacerbating pre-existing disparities. The practical lesson was clear: a healthcare system that marginalizes vulnerable populations ultimately compromises the health and safety of the entire nation.

The ethical and practical implications of inequality also intersect in the realm of policy. Efforts to address systemic disparities often face resistance rooted in ideological and economic arguments. Opponents of reform frequently cite the high costs of expanding access or express fears about government overreach, framing healthcare as a market commodity rather than a public good. Yet this perspective overlooks the long-term societal and economic costs of inaction. Addressing inequality is not just a moral imperative; it is a practical necessity for creating a healthier, more productive, and more cohesive society.

At the same time, proposed solutions must grapple with the complexities of the system itself. Simply redistributing resources or expanding coverage will not address deeper structural issues, such as the perverse incentives that drive up costs and prioritize profits. Ethical imperatives must be balanced with pragmatic strategies that align with the realities of a capitalist framework. For example, reform efforts might focus on incentivizing equitable practices within the private sector, fostering innovation that benefits underserved populations, or expanding programs like Medicaid while preserving market-driven efficiencies.

The persistence of inequality in the U.S. healthcare system poses a challenge to its legitimacy, forcing a reckoning with both its design and its values. Ethically, it demands a commitment to the principle that healthcare is a human right. Practically, it requires solutions that not only expand access but also address the root causes of disparity, from systemic racism to the profit motives entrenched in the system's structure. Bridging the gap between ethical aspirations and practical realities is no small task, but it is essential if the nation is to achieve a healthcare system that reflects its highest ideals while serving the needs of all its people.

CHAPTER 6: THE HUMAN COST OF PROFIT-DRIVEN CARE

He stood at the podium in a small community center, the lines of exhaustion etched deep into his face. Tom's voice trembled as he recounted how a single moment had unraveled his family's life. His wife, Karen, a healthy, vibrant mother of two, had suffered a ruptured appendix. It should have been a routine surgery, an inconvenience rather than a catastrophe. But the hospital was out of their insurance network, and the ambulance had taken her to the closest facility, one that didn't fall under their plan's coverage. What followed was a nightmare of denied claims, mounting bills, and endless appeals. Karen recovered, but the family did not.

"We had savings," Tom said, staring blankly at the floor. "We did everything right. But after the surgery, after the letters from the collection agencies started coming, it was like watching our life crumble in slow motion." The final blow came when their home, the one they had spent years saving for, was sold to cover the nearly $250,000 in medical debt. The room was silent, but Tom's story was not unique. He had come to the meeting because he'd heard others were going through the same thing—and he was right.

Around the country, millions of families face similar fates, their lives derailed by unexpected medical crises that leave them financially devastated. Despite having insurance, many Americans are just one emergency away from bankruptcy. In 2023, over 40% of U.S. adults reported carrying medical debt, and for a significant portion of them, the financial burden was insurmountable. Unlike in other developed nations, where healthcare is treated as a public good, Americans navigate a labyrinth of private insurers, opaque billing practices, and networks that seem designed to maximize profit rather than care.

For Karen and Tom, their story wasn't just about money; it was about betrayal. They had trusted the system to be there when they needed it most, only to find themselves crushed under its weight. It's a story that has become emblematic of a healthcare system where financial solvency, not medical need, determines outcomes. But the human cost isn't just limited to patients. Across the country, the same profit-driven structure that pushed Karen and Tom into bankruptcy is also burning out the very people tasked with delivering care: doctors, nurses, and frontline healthcare workers.

In an ER just hours away from Karen's home, a young nurse named Elena sits in her car after another grueling 12-hour shift, too exhausted to drive. She's 32, single, and has been a nurse for nearly a decade, but lately, she's begun to question how much longer she can continue. Her hospital, like many others, is understaffed, forcing her to take on more patients than she can safely handle. Each shift is a minefield of impossible decisions: who gets her attention first, the patient gasping for air or the elderly man showing signs of a heart attack? She often wonders if she's doing more harm than good.

Elena doesn't cry anymore; the tears dried up months ago. What she feels instead is something harder to name: a crushing guilt that no matter how hard she works, it's never enough. She knows the system isn't built to support her, just as it isn't built to support patients like Karen. And yet, she shows up each day, because the alternative feels even worse.

Karen and Elena's stories are not just anecdotes; they are symptoms of a larger disease. They illuminate a system that, for all its cutting-edge technology and medical innovation, is failing in its most basic purpose: to provide care. They are the human faces of a profit-driven machine, one that sacrifices well-being at every level—patients, providers, families—on the altar of financial gain. In a system like this, nobody emerges unscathed.

PATIENTS' STORIES—BANKRUPTCIES, MEDICAL DEBT, AND DELAYED CARE

When Anna Carter was diagnosed with breast cancer, she thought her insurance would shield her from financial ruin. She had worked for over 15 years as a teacher in a public school, diligently paying premiums for what she believed was comprehensive coverage. But as her treatment began, the bills started arriving. First, it was the out-of-pocket costs for chemotherapy, which her plan covered only partially. Then came the scans and biopsies, each carrying additional charges she hadn't anticipated. Finally, the denials—her insurer refused to approve a critical targeted therapy, labeling it as "experimental," despite her oncologist's insistence on its necessity. By the time Anna completed her treatment, she was cancer-free but drowning in $90,000 of medical debt. The stress of recovery was compounded by creditor calls and threats of legal action. Her once-perfect credit score plummeted, and she was forced to take on a second job tutoring after school to make minimum payments on her loans.

Anna's story is tragically common in the United States, where even those with insurance often find themselves financially gutted by medical emergencies.

Over 60% of all personal bankruptcies in the U.S. are tied to medical expenses, and studies consistently show that a majority of those bankruptcies involve individuals who were insured at the time of their illness or injury. It is a grim irony: the very coverage meant to protect against financial devastation often falls short when it is needed most. In a system designed to optimize profits, patients like Anna become collateral damage.

For others, the consequences of delayed or denied care can be far worse than financial hardship. Marcus Jennings, a 52-year-old truck driver from rural Alabama, knew something was wrong when the chest pain that had been nagging him for weeks worsened. He went to his local clinic, but with no insurance and a history of high blood pressure, he was told he'd need to pay upfront for further tests. He hesitated, unable to afford the $800 required for an echocardiogram. Three weeks later, Marcus collapsed in his driveway, clutching his chest. By the time paramedics arrived, it was too late. His wife later found the pamphlets on heart disease he'd brought home from the clinic, along with the notes he'd made about finding the money for the tests.

Stories like Marcus's reveal the stark disparities in access that define the U.S. healthcare system. For uninsured or underinsured patients, even minor health concerns can spiral into life-threatening conditions when delayed care is the only option. Studies show that uninsured individuals are three times more likely to delay or forgo care compared to those with coverage, and they are also more likely to die from preventable or treatable conditions. The system rewards those who can pay and punishes those who cannot, often with deadly consequences.

Even when care is accessible, the financial aftermath can stretch into every aspect of a patient's life. After his son's leukemia diagnosis, Javier Morales, a construction worker in Texas, spent months juggling medical appointments, insurance negotiations, and long hours on job sites to keep up with his family's mounting bills. Though his employer offered insurance, the high deductibles and out-of-pocket costs left him scrambling to cover even basic expenses. Javier sold his truck, drained his savings, and borrowed from relatives just to keep up with his son's treatment. By the time his son entered remission, Javier and his wife were living paycheck to paycheck, their financial stability shattered.

This is the paradox of the American healthcare system: it offers some of the most advanced treatments and technologies in the world but only to those who can afford them—or are willing to endure a lifetime of debt to access them. The system does not merely fail patients; it actively exploits them. Hospitals inflate prices, insurance companies deny claims, and pharmaceutical companies charge astronomical sums for life-saving drugs. The result is a healthcare landscape that is not a safety net but a minefield, where one wrong step can ruin lives.

These stories of medical debt, delayed care, and financial despair are not outliers. They are woven into the fabric of a system designed to prioritize profit over people. They expose the human toll of a model that commodifies care, leaving millions of Americans to navigate an unforgiving maze of bureaucracy, high costs, and financial precarity. For every Anna, Marcus, and Javier, there are countless others suffering silently, their struggles unseen but no less devastating. The cost of care in America is not just measured in dollars—it is measured in lives broken, opportunities lost, and futures stolen.

HEALTHCARE WORKERS—THE HIDDEN TOLL OF BURNOUT AND MORAL INJURY

In the dimly lit breakroom of a busy urban hospital, Dr. Sarah Collins sat with her head in her hands, the soft hum of vending machines the only sound breaking the silence. She had just come from the ICU, where she had to tell yet another family that there was nothing more they could do for their loved one. It wasn't the first time she had delivered such news, nor would it be the last. But this case had hit her differently. The patient, a 38-year-old father of three, had come in with complications from untreated diabetes. He'd skipped insulin doses for months after losing his job—and his health insurance.

"It didn't have to end this way," Sarah whispered to herself, her words heavy with frustration. She knew that with earlier intervention, he could have lived. But the system had failed him, and it was Sarah who now bore the burden of carrying his family's grief. As she stared at the untouched cup of coffee in front of her, she felt the familiar pangs of exhaustion, guilt, and helplessness—the steady erosion of her spirit that had begun years ago but now felt impossible to ignore.

For Sarah, and for countless other healthcare workers, the weight of practicing medicine in a profit-driven system is more than physical exhaustion; it is a deep, unrelenting moral injury. She entered medicine to save lives and heal, yet each day, she finds herself fighting a system that prioritizes financial gain over patient outcomes. Patients denied care, rushed discharges, insufficient staffing—each compromise chips away at her sense of purpose. The ideals that drew her to the field clash violently with the economic realities of a system designed to extract value rather than provide care.

Nurses like Elena Ramirez feel the same crushing weight. After years of working 12-hour shifts on a medical-surgical unit in a suburban hospital, Elena's compassion feels worn thin. She spends more time on paperwork than with her patients, forced to meet productivity quotas that dictate how many patients she must discharge each day. Her hospital, recently acquired by a private equity firm, implemented cost-cutting measures that eliminated support staff and increased her workload. She now routinely cares for twice the number of patients deemed safe, leaving her scrambling to prioritize care and make impossible decisions.

One night, after administering medication to an elderly patient recovering from surgery, Elena noticed the man's labored breathing. She wanted to stay longer to assess him, but her pager buzzed—a critical call from another room. Hours later, she returned to find the man in respiratory distress. Though the rapid response team stabilized him, Elena couldn't shake the feeling that she had failed him. That night, she sat in her car in the hospital parking lot, unable to start the engine, her hands trembling from the anxiety and guilt that had become her constant companions.

The toll on healthcare workers extends beyond burnout; it seeps into every corner of their lives. Studies show that physicians are at an alarmingly high risk of depression, with suicide rates significantly higher than those of the general population. Nurses, too, face staggering levels of mental health challenges, often exacerbated by chronic understaffing, workplace violence, and the emotional strain of watching preventable suffering unfold daily. Many healthcare workers report feeling trapped in a system that forces them to ration care, knowing that every cut corner, every delay, carries the potential to harm patients.

The profit-driven nature of the American healthcare system magnifies these pressures. Administrators often focus on metrics like bed turnover rates, billing codes, and reimbursement schedules, leaving little room for the humanity of care. Healthcare workers, caught in the middle, must reconcile their desire to provide quality care with the constant demands of efficiency and profitability. For many, this creates an unbearable sense of cognitive dissonance—a profound moral conflict between what they know is right for their patients and what the system allows them to do.

This unrelenting pressure has given rise to what experts call "moral injury," a condition distinct from burnout. Unlike burnout, which stems from overwork and exhaustion, moral injury arises when professionals are forced to act in ways that contradict their ethical beliefs. Healthcare workers like Sarah and Elena describe feeling powerless in the face of a system that often forces them to compromise on care due to financial constraints. These moments accumulate, creating a sense of guilt and betrayal that can linger for years.

The consequences are stark. Turnover rates among nurses and physicians are rising, with many leaving the profession altogether. Those who remain often do so out of a sense of duty but find themselves increasingly disconnected from the work they once loved. For patients, the impact is equally dire: when healthcare workers are stretched to their limits, care quality suffers, and mistakes become more frequent.

The human toll of this system is profound. It destroys not only the lives of patients but also the well-being of those entrusted to care for them. Healthcare workers like Sarah and Elena are the backbone of the system, yet they are too often treated as disposable resources, their compassion exploited and their resilience taken for granted. They bear the burden of a system that values profits over people, carrying the emotional scars long after the shifts end and the lights in the hospital corridors dim.

CONNECTING THE PATIENT AND WORKER EXPERIENCES

The stories of patients and healthcare workers in the U.S. healthcare system are not isolated tragedies; they are deeply intertwined, two sides of the same coin in a profit-driven model. For every patient crushed by insurmountable medical debt or denied critical care, there is a healthcare worker grappling with the moral fallout of their suffering. The system creates a chain reaction of harm: patients are left to navigate a labyrinth of costs, denials, and delays, while the very professionals tasked with their care are left powerless to intervene, forced to operate within the constraints of a system that prioritizes financial margins over human lives.

Consider Anna Carter's oncologist, the one who fought unsuccessfully to secure approval for the targeted therapy her cancer required. While Anna faced the financial devastation of her treatment, her doctor was caught in an endless loop of appeals, paperwork, and rejections from the insurance company. Despite years of training and expertise, the oncologist found her clinical judgment overridden by financial algorithms and actuarial tables. In a system designed to quantify care in terms of cost-effectiveness rather than outcomes, the physician became as much a victim of the system as her patient—though in a different way.

This mutual suffering reveals the perverse logic of a healthcare model that commodifies care. Patients are reduced to revenue streams, and providers are cast as cogs in an industrialized process, their decisions constrained by financial considerations far removed from the bedside. Doctors and nurses witness the ripple effects of the system daily: patients foregoing necessary medications, delaying treatments, or showing up in emergency rooms with advanced conditions that could have been treated months earlier. For healthcare workers, these moments are more than frustrations—they are emotional wounds that accumulate over time, leaving them disillusioned and demoralized.

When Marcus Jennings died of a heart attack after delaying care he couldn't afford, the local clinic staff that turned him away felt the echoes of his loss. The front-desk worker who informed him of the $800 upfront fee for testing wasn't responsible for the cost structure, yet she became the face of the system's indifference. The attending physician who briefly reviewed his case felt the weight of knowing Marcus needed urgent care but had no way to provide it without violating hospital policies. The grief that followed wasn't just felt by Marcus's family; it spread quietly through the clinic, another reminder to its staff of the limits imposed on their humanity.

For healthcare workers, the cumulative effect of these moments often leads to moral injury. When Elena Ramirez, the overburdened nurse in the understaffed hospital, was forced to prioritize one critical patient over another, she bore the weight of the decisions no caregiver should ever have to make. That night, when she returned to find her elderly patient in respiratory distress, it wasn't just an operational failure—it was a moment that etched itself into her memory, feeding her guilt and eroding her confidence in her ability to provide care. For every corner cut, every patient overlooked, workers like Elena carry the burden of a system they cannot change but cannot fully reconcile with their ethical responsibilities.

This connection between patient and worker is a vicious cycle. Patients who are failed by the system—through delayed care, denied treatments, or unaffordable bills—place greater strain on healthcare workers, who must then manage the consequences of those failures. At the same time, healthcare workers, stretched beyond their limits, cannot provide the level of care patients need, compounding the very issues they seek to resolve. Patients suffer in immediate, tangible ways: in pain that goes untreated, in diseases that progress unchecked, in lives that are cut short. Providers suffer in more insidious ways, their mental health fraying under the pressure of impossible expectations and ethical compromises.

The system pits patients and providers against one another in a way that obscures the true source of the dysfunction: the structural prioritization of profit over care. Patients, understandably, grow frustrated with overworked nurses or physicians who seem rushed or detached, unaware that those same workers are battling an unrelenting tide of administrative tasks, corporate demands, and staff shortages. Healthcare workers, meanwhile, find themselves drained of empathy, their compassion eroded by long hours and systemic inefficiencies, making it harder to connect with the patients who need them most.

At its most basic level, this dynamic exposes a profound betrayal of the social contract that should bind the healthcare system together. Patients enter the system seeking healing and support, while workers join the profession driven by a calling to help others. Yet both groups are left disillusioned, casualties of a system that forces them to compromise their needs and ideals. Their shared struggles, though often viewed in isolation, are inextricably linked, woven together by a system that treats care as a commodity rather than a human right.

The patient-worker relationship should be one of trust, empathy, and mutual support, but in the current system, it is too often defined by frustration, resentment, and shared helplessness. The cost of this fractured dynamic is not only personal but systemic, perpetuating a cycle of harm that deepens the inequities and inefficiencies at the heart of American healthcare. Until the connection between patient suffering and worker burnout is acknowledged and addressed, the system will continue to fail both groups, leaving behind a trail of broken lives and unmet promises.

The Broader Implications of a Profit-Driven System

The ripple effects of a profit-driven healthcare system extend far beyond the immediate struggles of patients and providers, shaping broader societal dynamics and reinforcing systemic inequalities. At its core, this model turns healthcare into an economic transaction, prioritizing financial viability over equitable access to care. In doing so, it undermines public trust, exacerbates social disparities, and compromises the very foundation of a system meant to serve as a safety net for all.

One of the most troubling implications is the erosion of the social fabric that binds communities together. Healthcare is not merely an individual concern; it is a public good that affects entire populations. When access to care is contingent upon one's financial status, the consequences ripple outward, creating stark divisions between those who can afford timely, quality treatment and those who cannot. Communities with concentrated poverty, often home to marginalized groups, face higher rates of chronic illness, shorter life expectancies, and lower overall health outcomes. These disparities feed into broader cycles of inequality, perpetuating economic disadvantages and social stratification.

Moreover, the profit motive introduces a troubling calculus into healthcare decision-making. Resources are disproportionately allocated to high-revenue services like elective procedures, specialty care, and cutting-edge technologies, often at the expense of essential, community-based services like primary care and mental health support. Rural hospitals, unable to sustain profitability in a system driven by economies of scale, are forced to close their doors, leaving vast swaths of the population without adequate access to care. In urban settings, the same logic manifests in healthcare deserts, where low-income neighborhoods are left with underfunded clinics and overburdened emergency rooms. This misalignment of priorities reveals a fundamental tension: the areas of greatest medical need are often the least financially lucrative, creating gaps in care that disproportionately harm the most vulnerable.

The profit-driven system also distorts the incentives for innovation and research. While the United States is undeniably a leader in medical advancements, the focus on marketable breakthroughs often sidelines efforts to address less glamorous but equally urgent public health challenges. Pharmaceutical companies, for instance, invest heavily in developing blockbuster drugs for conditions that promise high returns, such as chronic diseases prevalent in affluent populations, while neglecting treatments for rare diseases, tropical illnesses, or public health crises that predominantly affect poorer communities. This imbalance reflects a troubling truth: the value of innovation in American healthcare is too often measured by its profitability rather than its societal impact.

On a broader scale, the financialization of healthcare undermines public trust in the system. When patients view hospitals, insurance companies, and pharmaceutical firms as profit-seeking entities, skepticism replaces confidence, and fear supplants reassurance. Patients are left wondering whether their prescribed treatments are truly in their best interest or merely a means to maximize revenue. Healthcare workers, too, experience this erosion of trust, as their clinical expertise is overridden by corporate policies and bureaucratic mandates. The result is a pervasive sense of alienation: patients feel abandoned by the system, while providers feel estranged from their purpose.

This alienation has profound political consequences. Healthcare becomes a polarizing issue, a flashpoint for debates about the role of government, the limits of free-market principles, and the meaning of fairness in a capitalist society. Efforts to reform the system are stymied by entrenched interests and ideological divides, with proposed solutions often reflecting partisan priorities rather than a genuine commitment to improving outcomes. The Affordable Care Act, for example, sought to expand access to care but faced fierce opposition for its perceived encroachment on market freedoms. Conversely, conservative reforms aimed at reducing regulatory burdens are often criticized for prioritizing cost containment over comprehensive coverage. The result is a system locked in perpetual stalemate, unable to evolve in response to the needs of its population.

Perhaps most concerning is the way the profit-driven model reshapes cultural attitudes toward health and care. In a system where financial success is equated with moral worth, individuals are often blamed for their health outcomes, regardless of the structural barriers they face. Chronic illnesses are framed as failures of personal responsibility rather than the result of systemic inequities. This narrative not only stigmatizes the sick and the poor but also deflects attention from the deeper structural issues that perpetuate these conditions. It fosters a culture of individualism that obscures the collective nature of health, eroding the sense of shared responsibility that is essential to addressing public health challenges.

The broader implications of a profit-driven healthcare system, then, are not confined to hospitals or clinics—they touch every facet of society. From the perpetuation of inequality to the distortion of innovation, from the erosion of trust to the polarization of politics, the consequences are far-reaching and deeply entrenched. As the system continues to prioritize financial imperatives over human needs, it risks further entrenching a status quo that benefits the few at the expense of the many. Addressing these challenges requires not just technical fixes but a fundamental rethinking of the values that underpin American healthcare, shifting the focus from profit margins to the collective well-being of the nation.

Part 3: Politics, Policy, and Power

Chapter 7: Healthcare as a Political Battlefield

Healthcare in the United States exists at the complex intersection of politics, economics, and morality. As a cornerstone of societal well-being, it has always been a deeply political issue, shaped by the ideologies that govern the nation at any given time. The very nature of healthcare—concerned as it is with life, death, and human dignity—makes it a topic fraught with ethical dilemmas and competing priorities. At the heart of these debates lies a fundamental question: is healthcare a right or a privilege? The answer to this question, though seemingly philosophical, carries profound practical consequences, influencing how resources are allocated, policies are crafted, and lives are impacted.

In a capitalist democracy like the United States, healthcare policy reflects the tensions inherent in reconciling market principles with social responsibility. Progressive ideologies frame healthcare as a basic human right, an essential service that must be guaranteed by the state to ensure equity and justice. Conversely, conservative viewpoints emphasize personal responsibility and the efficiencies of free markets, arguing that government intervention distorts incentives and stifles innovation. These conflicting perspectives have not only defined the nation's healthcare landscape but have also fueled some of its most contentious political battles.

Policy decisions in healthcare are never made in a vacuum. They are shaped by the broader sociopolitical climate, economic constraints, and the influence of powerful stakeholders. The ideological fault lines between progressives and conservatives are evident in every aspect of the system, from debates over public insurance programs to disputes about the role of private enterprise. While progressives advocate for expanding government programs like Medicare and Medicaid to cover more Americans, conservatives argue that such initiatives lead to inefficiency, dependency, and unsustainable public spending. These positions are not merely abstract; they are embedded in legislative battles, public discourse, and the lived experiences of millions.

The polarization surrounding healthcare is further exacerbated by its status as both a deeply personal and profoundly collective issue. Few policy areas touch lives as intimately as healthcare does. It is not just a matter of economic calculation or political theory but one of survival and quality of life. Yet, the very intimacy of healthcare also makes it a fertile ground for ideological manipulation. Politicians on all sides use emotionally charged narratives to sway public opinion, often simplifying complex issues into binary choices that obscure the trade-offs involved.

In the United States, healthcare policy is not just shaped by the principles of fairness and access; it is also influenced by economic realities. The healthcare industry accounts for nearly a fifth of the nation's GDP, making it a powerful economic engine and a lucrative domain for various stakeholders. This dual character—as both a moral imperative and a market commodity—complicates any effort to find consensus. Balancing the competing demands of profit, access, and innovation requires navigating a labyrinth of conflicting interests, from insurance companies and pharmaceutical firms to hospitals, providers, and patients themselves.

The ideological divide in healthcare policy is not unique to the United States, but its manifestation here is particularly stark. Unlike many other developed nations, where there is a general consensus about the government's role in providing healthcare, the United States remains deeply divided. This division is not simply a matter of policy preferences but is rooted in the country's historical, cultural, and economic context. The result is a system that is both highly innovative and profoundly unequal, excelling in cutting-edge medical technologies while leaving millions without adequate care.

At the very center, the intersection of politics and healthcare reflects the nation's struggle to define its values and priorities. It is a microcosm of broader societal debates about the role of government, the ethics of profit, and the responsibilities of citizenship. The battles waged over healthcare policy are as much about identity and ideology as they are about budgets and benefits. These battles shape not only the structure of the healthcare system but also the lives of those who depend on it, making the political dimensions of healthcare inescapably human.

THE PROGRESSIVE VISION: HEALTHCARE AS A RIGHT

The progressive vision of healthcare rests on the belief that access to medical services is a fundamental human right, not a privilege dictated by socioeconomic status or geographic location. This perspective emphasizes equity and universality, advocating for a system in which every individual, regardless of their financial means, has access to essential care. Progressives view healthcare as a moral obligation of society, arguing that a just and compassionate nation cannot allow disparities in health outcomes to persist simply because of structural inequalities or economic barriers.

This vision draws from global examples, particularly the universal healthcare systems in countries like Canada, the United Kingdom, and Scandinavia, where government plays a central role in ensuring equitable access. In these nations, healthcare is seen as a public good, akin to education or infrastructure, and the government's role is to guarantee its availability through policies that prioritize collective well-being over individual profit. Progressives often point to these systems as evidence that universal coverage is not only morally right but also economically feasible, leading to better health outcomes at lower per capita costs.

In the United States, progressive advocacy for healthcare as a right has coalesced around calls for expansive reforms such as Medicare for All, which envisions a single-payer system eliminating private insurance in favor of universal public coverage. Proponents argue that this model would address the inefficiencies and inequities inherent in the current profit-driven system, which often leaves patients grappling with exorbitant costs and inconsistent access. By removing the profit motive from critical aspects of healthcare delivery, progressives contend, the system can focus on patient outcomes rather than shareholder returns.

The ideological foundation of this vision is rooted in the principle of social solidarity—the idea that society functions best when it collectively addresses its members' basic needs. Healthcare is framed as a common good, one that underpins not just individual well-being but also broader societal stability and productivity. Advocates argue that the current system, which allows millions to go uninsured or underinsured, creates ripple effects that harm everyone, from preventable illnesses that strain public resources to the economic inefficiencies of untreated conditions reducing workforce productivity.

Yet, the progressive vision faces significant challenges in implementation. Critics often point to the high costs associated with universal programs, raising concerns about tax increases and government inefficiency. Progressives counter these arguments by highlighting the inefficiencies of the current system, where administrative expenses, inflated pricing, and the complexity of private insurance drive costs far beyond those of universal systems abroad. They argue that reallocating resources from private profits to public investment would not only be equitable but also economically rational.

The Affordable Care Act (ACA), signed into law in 2010, represents a landmark effort to align the U.S. system closer to progressive ideals. While falling short of the single-payer model, the ACA expanded Medicaid, created insurance exchanges to improve access, and imposed regulations on insurers to prevent discriminatory practices. For many progressives, however, the ACA was a compromise rather than a solution—a step forward that left significant gaps in coverage and failed to address the fundamental issues of cost control and the profit-driven nature of the system.

Opposition to this vision is fierce, often fueled by ideological and financial interests. Critics argue that government involvement stifles innovation, reduces quality, and imposes undue burdens on taxpayers. Conservative policymakers and stakeholders in the private sector frame universal healthcare as a threat to individual freedom, emphasizing personal responsibility and market efficiency as superior mechanisms for distributing healthcare resources. The framing of healthcare as a right, they contend, risks undermining these values by prioritizing collective guarantees over individual choice.

Despite these criticisms, the progressive vision persists, driven by a growing awareness of the system's failings and the human cost of inaction. High-profile campaigns for Medicare for All and the rising prominence of healthcare reform in political discourse signal a shift in public attitudes, particularly among younger generations who are less tethered to traditional notions of market-based solutions. The progressive argument is not merely about policy but about redefining the ethical and social contract between citizens and their government, challenging the idea that healthcare is a commodity to be bought and sold rather than a service to be shared by all.

In this vision, the future of healthcare is not just a matter of fixing broken systems but of reimagining the very foundation on which they are built. It is a call to prioritize human dignity over profit margins, to invest in collective well-being as a measure of societal success, and to embrace the idea that access to care is not an entitlement but an inalienable right.

THE CONSERVATIVE PERSPECTIVE: HEALTHCARE AS PERSONAL RESPONSIBILITY

The conservative perspective on healthcare is deeply rooted in the principles of personal responsibility, limited government intervention, and free market solutions. Conservatives argue that healthcare, while essential, is not inherently a right but a service that individuals should access through personal effort, economic participation, and choice. This viewpoint frames healthcare as an outcome of individual responsibility and merit, emphasizing that citizens, rather than the state, should bear the primary burden of securing their health and well-being.

At the core of the conservative argument is a belief in market efficiency. Conservatives contend that the free market, when allowed to operate without excessive government interference, encourages innovation, competition, and cost control. They posit that healthcare functions best when it remains a product governed by supply and demand, where providers, insurers, and pharmaceutical companies compete to offer the best services at the lowest prices. Government intervention, in this view, distorts these market forces, leading to inefficiencies, inflated costs, and reduced quality of care.

One of the cornerstone policy approaches aligned with conservative values is the promotion of health savings accounts (HSAs) and high-deductible health plans. HSAs, which allow individuals to save money tax-free for medical expenses, are championed as tools for empowering consumers to make informed healthcare decisions. By encouraging patients to shop for value and make cost-conscious choices, conservatives argue that HSAs foster greater accountability and reduce unnecessary expenditures. In this model, healthcare spending is personalized, shifting the financial burden to individuals while reducing reliance on third-party payers.

The conservative approach also emphasizes the importance of decentralization. Conservatives advocate for state-level solutions to healthcare challenges, arguing that states are better equipped to address the specific needs of their populations than a one-size-fits-all federal policy. Programs like Medicaid, from this perspective, should be block-granted to states, giving local governments greater flexibility to design systems tailored to their demographics and budgets. This approach aligns with the broader conservative philosophy of federalism, which seeks to limit centralized power and enhance local governance.

The Affordable Care Act (ACA), often referred to as "Obamacare," has been a focal point of conservative criticism. Conservatives view the ACA's expansion of government oversight, mandates on individuals and employers, and establishment of insurance exchanges as antithetical to their principles. The individual mandate, in particular, was seen as an infringement on personal freedom, compelling citizens to purchase insurance regardless of their needs or financial situation. Repealing and replacing the ACA became a rallying cry for conservatives, culminating in numerous legislative attempts to dismantle or revise its provisions.

Instead of broad federal programs, conservatives favor policies that encourage private-sector solutions and individual participation. One example is the emphasis on short-term health plans, which offer lower-cost coverage with fewer benefits. While critics decry these plans for their limited scope, conservatives argue they provide affordable options for healthy individuals who do not require comprehensive coverage. Similarly, conservatives support reforms that reduce regulatory barriers for insurers, allowing them to sell plans across state lines and offer customized coverage packages.

Underlying these policy preferences is a philosophical commitment to the idea that over-reliance on government breeds dependency. Conservatives caution that expansive government healthcare programs, while well-intentioned, erode self-reliance, discourage personal health responsibility, and stifle innovation. They argue that when the state assumes the role of primary provider, individuals lose the incentive to maintain healthy lifestyles or manage their healthcare consumption prudently. Personal responsibility, in this view, is both a moral imperative and a practical necessity for sustaining a viable healthcare system.

Conservatives also raise concerns about the fiscal sustainability of large-scale government healthcare initiatives. Universal coverage programs, they argue, place unsustainable burdens on taxpayers, lead to higher deficits, and necessitate rationing of care. By keeping government involvement minimal and leveraging the efficiencies of the private sector, conservatives believe healthcare can remain affordable without sacrificing quality or innovation. They often point to the failures of single-payer systems in other countries, where long wait times, limited access to specialists, and bureaucratic inefficiencies are presented as cautionary tales.

Despite these convictions, the conservative perspective faces criticism for its perceived lack of compassion and inclusivity. Opponents argue that market-driven healthcare exacerbates inequalities, leaving vulnerable populations—such as the uninsured, the underinsured, and those with pre-existing conditions—without adequate protection. Conservatives counter this critique by highlighting the importance of safety nets for the truly needy, advocating for targeted subsidies and charity care to address gaps in the system without compromising market principles.

In this vision, healthcare is not framed as an entitlement but as a personal endeavor intertwined with broader economic participation. The conservative approach seeks to balance individual freedom with fiscal responsibility, prioritizing market-driven innovation and efficiency over collective guarantees. It reflects a broader ideological belief in the primacy of personal choice, the virtues of competition, and the dangers of government overreach. While its critics see it as prioritizing profit over people, its advocates view it as the most viable path to sustainable, high-quality healthcare that rewards responsibility and incentivizes innovation.

CASE STUDY 1: THE AFFORDABLE CARE ACT

The Affordable Care Act (ACA), often referred to as "Obamacare," stands as a defining moment in American healthcare policy, embodying a progressive vision of universal access to care through expanded government oversight. Passed in 2010 under the Obama administration, the ACA represented the most significant overhaul of the U.S. healthcare system since the establishment of Medicare and Medicaid in 1965. Its passage ignited intense political debate, as it challenged foundational assumptions about the role of government, the private sector, and individual responsibility in healthcare. Examining the ACA provides a lens into the broader ideological battles that define the healthcare landscape in the United States.

In its simplest form, the ACA aimed to address three pervasive issues in the American healthcare system: the lack of access to affordable insurance, the exclusion of individuals with pre-existing conditions, and the unsustainable rise in healthcare costs. To achieve these objectives, the legislation introduced several transformative measures. Among them was the individual mandate, a controversial provision requiring most Americans to maintain health insurance or face a tax penalty. This mandate sought to expand the risk pool by ensuring that both healthy and sick individuals participated in the insurance market, thereby mitigating adverse selection and stabilizing premiums.

Another cornerstone of the ACA was the expansion of Medicaid, the federal-state program that provides health coverage to low-income individuals. By broadening eligibility to include those earning up to 138% of the federal poverty level, the ACA brought millions of previously uninsured Americans into the healthcare system. This expansion was initially intended to be nationwide, but a 2012 Supreme Court ruling made Medicaid expansion optional for states, leading to a patchwork of coverage across the country. States that embraced expansion saw significant reductions in uninsured rates, while those that opted out faced persistent coverage gaps, particularly in rural and low-income communities.

The ACA also sought to increase affordability and accessibility through the establishment of health insurance marketplaces, or exchanges. These online platforms allowed individuals and small businesses to compare and purchase insurance plans, often with the assistance of federal subsidies based on income. For many Americans, these subsidies significantly reduced the cost of premiums, making coverage more attainable. However, critics argued that the exchanges imposed excessive regulatory burdens on insurers, limiting plan flexibility and driving some providers out of the market.

One of the most popular provisions of the ACA was its prohibition against denying coverage or charging higher premiums based on pre-existing conditions. Prior to the ACA, millions of Americans faced insurmountable barriers to obtaining insurance due to medical histories. By eliminating these exclusions, the ACA fundamentally reshaped the relationship between insurers and consumers, shifting the focus from risk assessment to universal inclusion. This provision, coupled with the mandate to cover essential health benefits such as preventive care, maternity services, and mental health treatment, represented a significant expansion of consumer protections.

Despite these achievements, the ACA faced fierce opposition from conservative lawmakers and advocacy groups, who viewed it as an overreach of federal authority. Critics contended that the individual mandate infringed on personal freedom, forcing individuals to purchase a product they may not want or need. Additionally, opponents argued that the ACA's regulatory requirements stifled competition and innovation in the insurance market, driving up costs for some consumers. Small businesses, in particular, expressed concerns about the employer mandate, which required companies with 50 or more full-time employees to offer health insurance or face penalties.

The fiscal implications of the ACA also became a point of contention. While proponents highlighted that the law was designed to be deficit-neutral, funded through a combination of taxes on high-income earners, fees on insurers, and cuts to Medicare spending, critics questioned its long-term sustainability. The

Cadillac tax, a levy on high-cost employer-sponsored plans, was particularly controversial and ultimately delayed and repealed due to bipartisan resistance.

The political battle over the ACA culminated in numerous attempts to repeal or weaken the law, particularly during the Trump administration. In 2017, a Republican-controlled Congress succeeded in eliminating the individual mandate penalty as part of the Tax Cuts and Jobs Act, effectively undermining one of the ACA's key mechanisms for maintaining market stability. Efforts to repeal the ACA in its entirety, however, failed to gain sufficient support, reflecting the complexity of dismantling a system that had become deeply embedded in the healthcare infrastructure.

The legacy of the ACA remains a subject of debate. On one hand, it expanded coverage to millions of Americans, reduced disparities in access to care, and established consumer protections that transformed the insurance market. On the other hand, it highlighted the deep ideological divides over the role of government in healthcare and exposed the limitations of a hybrid public-private system. For its supporters, the ACA represents a step toward the progressive ideal of healthcare as a right. For its detractors, it serves as a cautionary tale of government overreach and the unintended consequences of regulatory intervention.

Ultimately, the ACA illustrates the challenges of navigating the intersection of politics, economics, and healthcare. It underscores the difficulty of achieving universal access in a system that prioritizes market dynamics and individual choice. As the debate over healthcare reform continues, the ACA stands as both a milestone and a battleground, reflecting the complexities and contradictions of a deeply polarized nation.

CASE STUDY 2: CONSERVATIVE RESPONSES AND REFORMS

Conservative responses to healthcare reform in the United States, particularly in opposition to the Affordable Care Act (ACA), have been rooted in a philosophy emphasizing personal responsibility, market-based solutions, and a limited role for federal government intervention. These principles have shaped various policy proposals and reforms aimed at addressing the shortcomings of the healthcare system while avoiding what conservatives perceive as the ACA's overreach. Examining these responses reveals a distinct ideological framework that prioritizes individual choice, state autonomy, and fiscal discipline.

One of the most significant conservative counterpoints to the ACA was the proposed repeal-and-replace movement, which gained momentum during the Obama and Trump administrations. The effort sought to dismantle key components of the ACA, including the individual mandate, Medicaid expansion, and federal subsidies for insurance marketplaces. In their place, conservatives proposed reforms designed to lower costs and increase consumer choice without imposing federal mandates. While many of these efforts faced political and practical challenges, they illuminate core conservative strategies for healthcare reform.

A cornerstone of conservative policy has been the expansion of health savings accounts (HSAs), which allow individuals to save pre-tax dollars for medical expenses. HSAs are often paired with high-deductible health plans, incentivizing consumers to make cost-conscious decisions about their healthcare. Proponents argue that HSAs empower individuals by giving them direct control over their healthcare spending, fostering a sense of personal responsibility. Critics, however, contend that this approach disproportionately benefits higher-income individuals who can afford to contribute substantial amounts to their accounts while providing limited relief for those with lower incomes or chronic medical needs.

Another hallmark of conservative healthcare reform is the emphasis on deregulation to increase competition and reduce costs. For example, many proposals advocate for allowing the sale of health insurance across state lines, arguing that this would create a more competitive national marketplace. By eliminating state-specific mandates and regulations, conservatives believe insurers could offer more affordable and customizable plans. Opponents caution that this approach could lead to a "race to the bottom," where insurers base operations in states with the least stringent regulations, potentially undermining consumer protections.

Block grants and per-capita caps for Medicaid represent another key conservative reform strategy. Under the ACA, Medicaid expansion significantly increased federal funding to states to cover a broader population. Conservative proposals, however, seek to transition Medicaid to a block grant or capped funding model, giving states greater flexibility to design their programs while limiting federal spending. Supporters argue that this approach encourages innovation and efficiency at the state level, as states can tailor programs to meet their unique needs. Critics, however, warn that such reforms could lead to reduced benefits or eligibility as states grapple with funding constraints, exacerbating disparities in access to care.

Conservative reforms have also focused on addressing high prescription drug costs, though typically through market-based mechanisms rather than price controls. Proposals have included promoting greater transparency in drug pricing, increasing the use of generic and biosimilar medications, and streamlining the Food and Drug Administration's (FDA) approval process to bring new drugs to market more quickly. While these measures aim to leverage market competition to drive down costs, they often stop short of imposing direct government intervention, such as allowing Medicare to negotiate drug prices—a policy strongly opposed by many conservatives.

The Trump administration's healthcare policies provide a concrete example of conservative responses in action. In addition to the repeal of the individual mandate penalty through the Tax Cuts and Jobs Act of 2017, the administration introduced short-term, limited-duration insurance plans as an alternative to ACA-compliant plans. These plans were marketed as more affordable options for healthy individuals but were criticized for offering limited coverage and excluding protections for pre-existing conditions. The administration also sought to expand association health plans, allowing small businesses and self-employed individuals to band together to purchase insurance, potentially lowering costs but raising concerns about fragmented risk pools and reduced consumer protections.

Perhaps the most notable conservative healthcare reform proposal in recent years was the Graham-Cassidy bill, introduced in 2017. This legislation sought to repeal the ACA's Medicaid expansion and replace federal subsidies with block grants to states, giving them broad discretion over how to allocate funds. The bill also proposed eliminating the individual and employer mandates, emphasizing a shift away from federal requirements toward state-led innovation. While the bill garnered support among conservative lawmakers, it ultimately failed to pass due to concerns about its potential impact on coverage and access.

Conservative healthcare reforms have not been without criticism, even among their intended beneficiaries. Skeptics argue that the emphasis on market-based solutions and deregulation can lead to fragmented and inequitable outcomes, with the most vulnerable populations—low-income individuals, rural residents, and those with chronic conditions—bearing the brunt of reduced access and affordability. Furthermore, the focus on reducing federal spending often translates into difficult trade-offs for states, insurers, and providers, creating challenges in maintaining comprehensive care.

Despite these critiques, conservative responses to healthcare reform reflect a consistent ideological commitment to individual autonomy, fiscal prudence, and decentralized governance. They offer an alternative vision to progressive approaches, one that prioritizes empowering consumers, fostering competition, and limiting government intervention. However, the practical implementation of these reforms remains a complex and contentious endeavor, as policymakers grapple with balancing cost containment, access, and quality in an inherently fragmented healthcare system.

The political and ideological tensions surrounding conservative healthcare reforms underscore the broader challenge of achieving consensus on the future of American healthcare. While progressives and conservatives share a common goal of improving the system, their fundamentally different visions for how to achieve that goal continue to fuel debate and shape the trajectory of healthcare policy in the United States. The case of conservative reforms illustrates not only the ideological divide but also the enduring complexity of reconciling competing priorities in a deeply polarized environment.

The Role of Polarization in Shaping Healthcare Debates

The intensifying polarization of American politics has left few areas untouched, and healthcare policy has emerged as one of the most contentious battlegrounds. While disagreements about healthcare have long existed, the deep ideological divide in contemporary politics has transformed these debates into symbolic struggles over identity, values, and the role of government in society. This polarization has fundamentally shaped how healthcare policy is formulated, debated, and implemented, often prioritizing political gains over practical solutions.

Healthcare policy has become a litmus test for broader ideological commitments, with each side viewing its stance as a core expression of its values. For progressives, healthcare is framed as a universal right, emblematic of a society that prioritizes collective welfare and equity. On the other hand, conservatives approach healthcare as a matter of personal responsibility and market efficiency, seeing government overreach as a threat to individual freedoms. These starkly contrasting worldviews not only influence policy proposals but also deepen the divisions between political leaders and their constituencies.

One consequence of polarization is that healthcare policy discussions often devolve into zero-sum battles, where compromise is seen as betrayal. The Affordable Care Act (ACA) serves as a prime example. Initially conceived with bipartisan elements—drawing on ideas from earlier conservative proposals—the ACA was ultimately passed without a single Republican vote in Congress. Its association with the Democratic Party and President Obama rendered it a symbol of progressive governance in the eyes of conservatives, solidifying partisan opposition. Efforts to repeal or undermine the ACA, such as the legal challenges that reached the Supreme Court and the repeated repeal votes in Congress, became rallying points for conservative lawmakers, regardless of the policy's tangible effects.

Polarization also shapes public perceptions of healthcare reforms. Partisan media amplify and entrench ideological divisions, presenting healthcare policies not as nuanced solutions but as victories or threats to their respective audiences. For instance, progressive outlets often highlight the human cost of conservative reforms, such as reduced Medicaid coverage or limited protections for pre-existing conditions, casting them as morally untenable. Conversely, conservative media frequently frame progressive healthcare proposals as steps toward socialism, emphasizing the potential for increased taxes, inefficiencies, and government overreach.

This dynamic complicates the policymaking process, as public opinion becomes increasingly aligned with partisan identity rather than policy specifics. Surveys have shown that individuals' support or opposition to healthcare policies often correlates more strongly with their political affiliation than with their personal experiences or understanding of the policies. For example, while many provisions of the ACA—such as protections for pre-existing conditions—enjoy broad bipartisan support when discussed in isolation, the law as a whole remains divisive due to its partisan branding.

The role of polarization is further evident in the fragmented approach to healthcare across states. Republican-led states have frequently resisted federal healthcare initiatives like Medicaid expansion under the ACA, even when doing so would bring significant financial benefits and improve access to care for their residents. This resistance reflects not only ideological opposition to federal intervention but also the political calculus of opposing policies associated with the opposing party. Similarly, Democratic-led states have pursued more ambitious reforms, such as establishing public options or expanding subsidies, using healthcare policy as a platform to showcase progressive governance. The result is a patchwork system where access to and quality of care increasingly depend on one's geographic location and the prevailing political climate in that state.

Polarization also affects how healthcare crises are managed. The COVID-19 pandemic starkly illustrated how political divisions can hinder coordinated responses. From the outset, debates over mask mandates, vaccine distribution, and public health measures were infused with partisan rhetoric. Conservative leaders and media often framed these measures as infringements on personal liberty, while progressives emphasized collective responsibility and the role of science in guiding policy. This polarization not only shaped policy responses but also influenced public behavior, with vaccination rates and adherence to public health guidelines varying significantly along partisan lines.

The legislative gridlock fueled by polarization has broader implications for healthcare policy. Ambitious reforms, such as the implementation of a single-payer system or comprehensive cost-control measures, face steep obstacles in a divided Congress. Even incremental changes often become mired in partisan disputes, delaying or diluting potential progress. This paralysis perpetuates many of the systemic challenges in the healthcare system, from rising costs to inequities in access, leaving millions of Americans to bear the burden.

Yet, polarization does not solely obstruct progress; it also drives innovation in some instances. Competing visions for healthcare have spurred states to experiment with diverse approaches, providing valuable case studies for future reform. For example, conservative states have piloted initiatives emphasizing market-based solutions, such as work requirements for Medicaid recipients, while progressive states have explored pathways to universal coverage. While these experiments reflect divergent ideologies, they contribute to the broader understanding of what works and what doesn't in addressing complex healthcare challenges.

Ultimately, the role of polarization in shaping healthcare debates underscores the difficulty of achieving consensus in a deeply divided society. The intractable ideological divide often obscures the shared goal of improving the healthcare system, turning policy debates into symbolic contests rather than opportunities for constructive problem solving. For policymakers and advocates seeking to navigate this polarized landscape, the challenge lies in finding common ground that transcends partisan identity, focusing instead on practical solutions that resonate with the shared experiences and needs of the American people.

This task is not without precedent. Historical moments of bipartisan cooperation, such as the creation of Medicare and Medicaid in the 1960s, demonstrate that meaningful progress is possible even in times of political division. However, such achievements require political will, public trust, and a willingness to engage in good-faith negotiations—qualities that seem increasingly elusive in the current environment. As healthcare remains a central issue for voters and policymakers alike, the question of whether polarization can be bridged to address systemic challenges will continue to define the future of American healthcare.

THE GLOBAL CONTEXT: COMPARING IDEOLOGICAL APPROACHES

The global landscape of healthcare provides a rich context for understanding how ideological frameworks shape healthcare systems and outcomes. Across the world, nations adopt policies that reflect their historical, cultural, and political ideologies, offering valuable insights into the benefits and limitations of different approaches. Comparing these systems illuminates the influence of ideological underpinnings on accessibility, equity, and efficiency, and provides a lens through which the American healthcare debate can be viewed.

In countries where the ethos of collective responsibility predominates, healthcare is often treated as a universal right. Systems such as those in Canada, the United Kingdom, and the Nordic countries prioritize equitable access to care, financed primarily through taxation. These single-payer or heavily regulated systems embody the progressive vision that views healthcare as a fundamental public good. While critics of these models often cite challenges such as wait times for non-emergency services and constrained provider autonomy, their proponents highlight the absence of medical bankruptcies, lower administrative costs, and more equitable health outcomes as evidence of their effectiveness.

In stark contrast, market-driven systems like those in the United States emphasize individual responsibility and consumer choice, aligning with a more conservative ideological framework. The American model, characterized by its reliance on private insurance and employer-sponsored coverage, underscores the role of competition and innovation in driving quality and efficiency. Proponents argue that the system's flexibility fosters groundbreaking advancements in pharmaceuticals, medical devices, and specialized care. However, this approach also results in significant disparities, with millions of

Americans facing financial barriers to access and outcomes that lag behind those of other developed nations in key health metrics.

Hybrid systems, such as those in Germany, France, and Japan, straddle the ideological divide by blending public and private elements. These nations often achieve universal coverage through mandatory insurance schemes that integrate private providers with robust public oversight. For instance, Germany's system combines employer-based and government-subsidized insurance while maintaining strong regulatory controls to ensure affordability and equity. These mixed models demonstrate that ideological compromises can lead to systems that balance innovation with access, offering lessons for nations grappling with the tensions between market efficiency and social equity.

Developing countries provide yet another perspective, where healthcare systems are frequently shaped by resource constraints and external influences. In nations like India and Brazil, public health initiatives coexist with a burgeoning private sector, creating a dual system that reflects both the aspirations of universal care and the realities of limited infrastructure. The challenges faced by these countries—ranging from underfunded public facilities to the dominance of private out-of-pocket spending—highlight the importance of context in determining how ideological visions translate into policy.

A critical distinction between these global systems and the United States is the degree of political consensus surrounding healthcare. In many countries, even those with deep political divides, healthcare reforms often enjoy broad support as part of a shared commitment to public welfare. For example, Japan's universal healthcare system, implemented in the 1960s, has endured despite shifts in political leadership, reflecting a cultural consensus that prioritizes health as a national asset. Similarly, in Australia, reforms to expand access, such as the introduction of Medicare, were achieved through bipartisan collaboration, cementing the system's durability.

The lack of such consensus in the United States has perpetuated a fragmented and polarized approach to healthcare policy. While other nations debate refinements to their systems within a framework of agreed principles, American debates often return to foundational questions about the role of government, markets, and individual responsibility. This ideological impasse not only hinders comprehensive reform but also exacerbates the inequities and inefficiencies that characterize the current system.

Despite these differences, the global context also reveals common challenges that transcend ideological divides. Rising healthcare costs, aging populations, and the increasing prevalence of chronic diseases strain even the most robust systems, forcing nations to confront difficult trade-offs. Countries with universal systems grapple with budgetary pressures and the sustainability of funding mechanisms, while market-driven systems like the United States face mounting criticism for their inequities and inefficiencies. These shared challenges underscore the importance of looking beyond ideological debates to identify practical solutions that can address systemic issues.

The global response to the COVID-19 pandemic offers a poignant illustration of how ideological frameworks shape healthcare resilience. Countries with universal systems were often better equipped to implement coordinated responses, leveraging centralized public health infrastructures to manage testing, treatment, and vaccination efforts. In contrast, nations with fragmented systems faced significant hurdles in ensuring equitable access and coherence in their responses. Yet, the pandemic also highlighted the importance of innovation and adaptability, qualities often associated with market-driven systems. The rapid development of vaccines, led by companies in the United States and other market-oriented economies, showcased the potential of public-private collaboration in addressing global health crises.

For the United States, examining global models offers both cautionary tales and sources of inspiration. While it is unlikely that the American system will converge entirely with any single model, elements from other nations can inform efforts to balance competing priorities. For example, adopting mechanisms to reduce administrative overhead, such as standardized billing systems, could draw from the efficiencies of single-payer models. Similarly, policies to incentivize preventive care and address social determinants of health could emulate approaches seen in countries with strong public health traditions.

Ultimately, the global context underscores that healthcare systems are not merely technical constructs but reflections of societal values and priorities. The choices nations make about healthcare policy—whether to emphasize equity, efficiency, or innovation—are deeply influenced by their political and cultural landscapes. For the United States, the challenge lies in navigating its polarized ideological terrain to craft a system that aligns with its unique context while learning from the successes and failures of other nations. By recognizing healthcare as a shared human endeavor rather than a purely political issue, there is potential to move beyond entrenched divisions and toward a system that better serves all Americans.

THE HUMAN IMPACT OF POLITICAL BATTLES

Behind every political battle over healthcare lies the undeniable reality of human lives shaped, altered, or constrained by the decisions of policymakers. For individuals and families, the human impact of these ideological conflicts manifests in the most personal ways: through denied treatments, unmanageable medical bills, delayed care, or, conversely, lifesaving interventions enabled by systemic reforms. While the political discourse often frames healthcare in abstract terms—cost curves, market dynamics, or regulatory frameworks—it is the stories of those caught in the crossfire that reveal the true stakes of the debate.

For many Americans, the politicization of healthcare means living in a state of uncertainty. Patients with chronic conditions, for example, face immense pressure to navigate an ever-changing system. One year, they might have access to affordable medications through expanded Medicaid or marketplace subsidies; the next, a shift in political leadership could lead to cuts in funding or reduced benefits. This constant flux imposes not only financial strain but also emotional distress, as individuals struggle to plan for their health needs in an unpredictable environment.

Consider the plight of families who depend on programs like the Children's Health Insurance Program (CHIP). For years, CHIP has provided a safety net for children in low-income households, yet its funding has frequently become a bargaining chip in broader political negotiations. In moments of legislative gridlock, parents are left to wonder whether their children's access to essential care will continue, their sense of security eroded by the vicissitudes of partisan conflict. For these families, healthcare is not merely a policy issue but a daily reality that dictates their ability to protect and provide for their loved ones.

The human cost of political battles is also starkly evident in the experiences of those with pre-existing conditions. Before the implementation of the Affordable Care Act, insurers routinely denied coverage or charged exorbitant premiums to individuals with health histories deemed high-risk. For people like cancer survivors, individuals with diabetes, or those managing mental health conditions, this exclusion created insurmountable barriers to care. The ACA's provisions to protect these populations marked a watershed moment, yet they remain at risk of reversal as political factions continue to debate the law's merits. Each legal challenge to the ACA renews fears among these vulnerable groups, highlighting how deeply intertwined their wellbeing is with the ideological tides of the nation.

Healthcare workers, too, bear the brunt of these political conflicts. Physicians, nurses, and administrators often find themselves in the untenable position of reconciling their commitment to patient care with the constraints imposed by policy decisions. When funding cuts lead to staffing shortages, when regulatory shifts increase administrative burdens, or when patients delay care due to financial concerns, providers must navigate the ethical dilemmas that arise from a system shaped by political discord. Burnout, already a pervasive issue in the healthcare sector, is exacerbated by the added pressures of working within a politically charged environment where decisions at the legislative level ripple through every layer of the system.

Moreover, the ideological divide in healthcare policy perpetuates systemic inequities, with disproportionate impacts on marginalized communities. Racial and socioeconomic disparities in health outcomes, already entrenched by historical injustices, are further exacerbated by policies that prioritize market mechanisms over public investment. For communities with limited access to providers, affordable coverage, or public health resources, the political battles over healthcare are not academic exercises but existential threats. These disparities highlight a fundamental tension in the debate: while one ideological camp argues for efficiency and individual responsibility, the other emphasizes equity and collective welfare. For those on the losing side of these debates, the consequences are often devastating.

The politicization of healthcare also affects the broader social fabric, fueling polarization and eroding trust in institutions. When public health initiatives become entangled in partisan conflicts, the ability to mobilize collective action diminishes. The COVID-19 pandemic starkly illustrated this dynamic, as debates over mask mandates, vaccination campaigns, and emergency funding became battlegrounds for competing ideologies. Public health officials, once trusted as neutral experts, found themselves vilified by factions skeptical of government intervention, undermining efforts to achieve widespread compliance with lifesaving measures. The long-term repercussions of this erosion of trust extend beyond the pandemic, jeopardizing the capacity of the healthcare system to respond to future crises.

Yet amidst these challenges, stories of resilience and advocacy emerge, offering hope for a path forward. Patient advocacy groups, community health organizations, and grassroots movements have mobilized to counteract the human toll of political battles, amplifying the voices of those most affected. From campaigns to preserve Medicaid expansion to efforts to reduce prescription drug costs, these initiatives demonstrate the power of collective action to challenge entrenched interests and drive change. While progress is often incremental, these movements underscore the importance of centering the human experience in the healthcare debate, reframing the conversation from one of partisan conflict to one of shared responsibility.

Ultimately, the human impact of political battles over healthcare serves as both a cautionary tale and a call to action. As policymakers and stakeholders grapple with the complexities of reform, they must contend with the real-world consequences of their decisions, recognizing that healthcare is not merely a commodity or a policy issue but a cornerstone of human dignity. By prioritizing the needs of patients, providers, and communities, there is an opportunity to transcend ideological divides and create a system that honors the fundamental promise of healthcare: to alleviate suffering and promote wellbeing for all.

Towards a Pragmatic Path Forward

As the healthcare system in the United States continues to grapple with political polarization, economic pressures, and an ever-evolving landscape of technological advancements, the need for a pragmatic, balanced path forward has never been more urgent. The goal must be to create a system that can accommodate the complex needs of the population while addressing the realities of budget constraints, market forces, and political feasibility. A pragmatic path forward requires an acknowledgment of the strengths and limitations of both public and private models and a willingness to forge solutions that blend innovation, efficiency, and equity.

The first step in forging a pragmatic path forward is recognizing the importance of healthcare as a public good, even within the confines of a market-driven economy. Healthcare cannot and should not be treated solely as a commodity to be bought and sold; it is, at its core, a basic need that underpins the very fabric of society. At the same time, however, the realities of capitalism in the United States necessitate an approach that balances public and private involvement. This means embracing a hybrid model that allows for competition and innovation within a regulated framework, ensuring that the needs of all individuals are met, regardless of their ability to pay.

A pragmatic healthcare system must prioritize universal access to care while also addressing the concerns of those who believe that government intervention should be limited. It is not about choosing between one ideological extreme or another, but rather finding a middle ground that maximizes both equity and efficiency. For example, expanding access to affordable insurance through public options, like a robust Medicaid or Medicare for All model, could provide a foundation for healthcare equity, while allowing private insurers and providers to coexist in a competitive marketplace.

Such an approach would allow individuals to choose between public and private plans based on their personal preferences, while ensuring that no one is excluded from care due to financial constraints.

At the same time, the role of technology in healthcare cannot be ignored. Innovation in telemedicine, data analytics, and artificial intelligence has the potential to revolutionize care delivery, making it more efficient, personalized, and accessible. However, these advancements must be deployed thoughtfully to avoid exacerbating existing inequalities. For instance, while telemedicine can increase access to care for rural populations, it must also be accompanied by efforts to ensure broadband access and digital literacy for underserved communities. Similarly, the use of data-driven care models must be carefully regulated to protect patient privacy and prevent discrimination based on pre-existing conditions or socioeconomic status.

Another critical component of a pragmatic path forward is reforming the pharmaceutical industry to better balance innovation with affordability. The rising cost of prescription drugs remains one of the most significant burdens on the healthcare system, with life-saving medications often priced out of reach for many Americans. Addressing this issue requires a multi-pronged approach, including greater transparency in pricing, the elimination of drug price gouging, and the introduction of stronger price controls for certain essential medications. At the same time, incentives for research and development must remain strong to encourage continued innovation, especially in the development of new treatments for rare and complex conditions. A pragmatic solution would strike a balance between ensuring access to affordable medications and maintaining the economic incentives necessary for pharmaceutical companies to innovate.

Perhaps one of the most significant obstacles to reform is the political gridlock that has hindered progress for decades. The ideological divide between those who advocate for a more market-driven, individual responsibility approach to healthcare and those who push for a more expansive, government-run model has created an environment where compromise seems almost impossible. Yet, it is precisely through compromise that meaningful change can be achieved.

Politicians on both sides of the aisle must be willing to set aside partisan interests and work toward pragmatic solutions that address the needs of the American people. This means moving beyond symbolic gestures or superficial reforms and focusing on the real, tangible changes that can improve the lives of millions.

One such solution could involve a gradual move toward universal coverage through incremental reforms, such as expanding Medicaid in all states, increasing subsidies for the Affordable Care Act, and creating a public option that offers an affordable insurance alternative for those who are left out of the private insurance market. By gradually building toward a more inclusive system, policymakers can ensure that the transition is manageable and that the concerns of both progressives and conservatives are addressed. Additionally, such a phased approach would allow for the continuous evaluation and adjustment of policies based on real-world outcomes, making it easier to identify and address potential issues before they become insurmountable.

A pragmatic path forward must recognize the importance of personal responsibility in healthcare. While systemic reforms are necessary, individuals also have a role to play in improving their own health and wellbeing. Public health campaigns, education on prevention, and programs that encourage healthy lifestyles are essential components of any long-term healthcare strategy. By promoting wellness and preventative care, the overall burden on the healthcare system can be reduced, ensuring that resources are directed toward those who need them most.

The path to a better healthcare system in the United States does not lie in embracing extremes but in finding a middle ground that can accommodate the needs of all Americans. By focusing on practical solutions, such as expanding access, improving affordability, fostering innovation, and addressing political polarization, the U.S. can move toward a healthcare system that works for everyone. The goal is not to create a perfect system but a system that is effective, sustainable, and fair—one that prioritizes the health and wellbeing of all citizens, regardless of their income, background, or political affiliation.

Chapter 8: The Lobbyists' Playground

The United States healthcare system operates within one of the most heavily lobbied sectors in the country, a distinction that underscores the immense power wielded by corporate and industry stakeholders in shaping the policies that govern it. Lobbying in healthcare has become not just a tool for influence but a structural feature of the system itself, deeply embedded in how decisions are made, laws are crafted, and priorities are set. The scale of this influence is staggering, with billions of dollars spent annually by insurers, pharmaceutical companies, hospital associations, and medical device manufacturers to advocate for their interests at every level of government. The effect of this lobbying goes far beyond mere persuasion; it actively defines the contours of healthcare policy, often privileging corporate objectives over public health goals.

The historical trajectory of healthcare lobbying in the United States reveals its growing sophistication and reach. Early efforts were relatively modest, focused primarily on narrow, industry-specific concerns, such as securing favorable reimbursement rates or opposing regulations deemed burdensome. However, the mid-20th century brought a seismic shift as healthcare became increasingly central to federal and state governance. The creation of Medicare and Medicaid in the 1960s marked a turning point, introducing vast new funding streams that attracted heightened attention from industry players. Lobbying efforts quickly scaled up to influence the rules surrounding these programs, ensuring that private entities could carve out lucrative roles within publicly funded systems.

As the healthcare system expanded, so too did the complexity of the lobbying apparatus. Trade organizations like America's Health Insurance Plans (AHIP), the Pharmaceutical Research and Manufacturers of America (PhRMA), and the American Hospital Association (AHA) emerged as powerful entities capable of coordinating industry-wide efforts. These groups consolidated the voices of their respective sectors, allowing them to present a unified front when lobbying lawmakers and regulators. The resources at their disposal became formidable, enabling them to deploy armies of lobbyists, fund detailed policy research, and launch sophisticated public relations campaigns aimed at shaping public opinion.

The sheer volume of healthcare lobbying eclipses that of nearly every other sector, including defense, technology, and finance. In some years, healthcare expenditures on lobbying have accounted for more than 15% of all federal lobbying dollars, a testament to the stakes involved. These expenditures are not limited to direct lobbying activities but also include campaign contributions, funding for think tanks, and support for advocacy organizations that align with industry objectives. Such efforts ensure that healthcare stakeholders maintain a constant presence in the corridors of power, exerting influence on legislative processes long before bills reach the floor for debate.

What sets healthcare lobbying apart is its unparalleled ability to affect the lives of ordinary Americans. Unlike lobbying in other industries, which may focus on regulatory or tax issues with more diffuse impacts, healthcare lobbying touches directly on questions of access, affordability, and quality of care. The policies shaped by these efforts determine who receives treatment, how much it costs, and under what conditions care is delivered. This dynamic creates a profound tension between the profit motives of industry stakeholders and the ethical imperatives of ensuring equitable health outcomes. As healthcare continues to consume an ever-growing share of the national economy, this tension has only deepened, raising fundamental questions about whose interests are truly served by the system as it stands.

Lobbying in healthcare also operates through a revolving door that blurs the lines between industry and government. Former lawmakers and regulators frequently transition into high-paying lobbying roles, leveraging their insider knowledge and connections to advocate for industry interests. This revolving door not only amplifies the power of healthcare lobbyists but also creates an environment in which public policy can be unduly shaped by private gain. Critics argue that this dynamic undermines the integrity of the policymaking process, making it harder to achieve reforms that prioritize public health over corporate profits.

While the influence of healthcare lobbying is undeniable, it is not monolithic. Competing interests within the industry often result in battles over policy priorities, with insurers, pharmaceutical companies, and hospitals each vying to protect their own bottom lines. These internal conflicts can complicate legislative efforts, as lawmakers are frequently caught in the crossfire of competing lobbying campaigns. At the same time, the immense resources of these stakeholders often enable them to outmaneuver countervailing forces, such as consumer advocacy groups or public health organizations, which typically operate with far fewer resources.

The magnitude of healthcare lobbying underscores its role as both a symptom and a driver of the system's dysfunctions. On one hand, lobbying reflects the inherent complexity of a system in which public and private interests are deeply intertwined. On the other hand, it perpetuates a status quo in which meaningful reform becomes exceedingly difficult to achieve. The question of how to reconcile the legitimate need for industry input with the broader imperative of serving the public good remains a central challenge for policymakers. As the healthcare system faces mounting pressures, from rising costs to demographic shifts and technological disruptions, the influence of lobbying will undoubtedly continue to shape its evolution in profound and often contentious ways.

The Insurance Industry's Strategic Maneuvers

The insurance industry occupies a uniquely influential position within the healthcare landscape, serving as both a gatekeeper to medical access and a dominant force in shaping legislative and regulatory frameworks. This dual role allows insurers to wield tremendous power, not only in determining the terms under which care is provided but also in crafting policies that often protect their financial interests. Through sophisticated lobbying strategies and substantial financial investments, the insurance industry has entrenched itself as an indispensable stakeholder, strategically maneuvering to maintain and expand its influence.

One of the most effective tools at the disposal of the insurance industry is its ability to frame healthcare policy debates in ways that align with its priorities. By positioning themselves as critical intermediaries that ensure cost efficiency and patient protection, insurers have successfully cultivated an image of indispensability. This narrative often emphasizes their role in managing risk, controlling healthcare expenditures, and negotiating with providers to secure favorable pricing. However, behind this public-facing rhetoric lies a calculated effort to steer the policymaking process toward outcomes that safeguard their profit margins, often at the expense of broader systemic reforms.

The insurance industry's lobbying efforts are among the most extensive and well-coordinated in the healthcare sector. Trade organizations like America's Health Insurance Plans (AHIP) and the Blue Cross Blue Shield Association play central roles in these efforts, pooling resources to fund lobbying campaigns that target lawmakers, regulators, and the public. These campaigns often deploy a mix of direct lobbying, public relations strategies, and financial contributions to political candidates who are sympathetic to the industry's goals. By cultivating strong relationships with policymakers, insurers are able to exert substantial influence over the development of legislation and regulations that impact their operations.

A notable example of the insurance industry's strategic maneuvering can be observed in its response to the Affordable Care Act (ACA). While publicly supporting certain provisions of the ACA, such as the individual mandate, insurers simultaneously lobbied aggressively to shape the law in ways that favored their interests. They successfully pushed for the inclusion of provisions that guaranteed a steady influx of customers, such as subsidies for low-income individuals purchasing insurance on the exchanges, while also resisting measures that would have imposed stricter regulations on premium increases. This dual approach highlights the industry's ability to navigate complex legislative processes, securing concessions that enhance profitability while minimizing potential risks.

The insurance industry's influence extends beyond the federal level to state governments, where many key decisions about healthcare policy are made. State insurance commissioners, who are often elected or appointed with significant input from industry stakeholders, play a pivotal role in overseeing the industry. Insurers have been adept at lobbying state officials to shape regulations on issues such as network adequacy, premium rates, and coverage requirements. By leveraging their local presence and economic impact, insurers often succeed in framing their priorities as aligned with state interests, further entrenching their power.

Another critical aspect of the insurance industry's strategy is its use of data and analytics to bolster its lobbying efforts. Insurers possess vast troves of information on healthcare utilization, costs, and outcomes, which they use to support their policy positions. By commissioning studies, funding research, and collaborating with academic institutions, insurers can produce evidence that reinforces their narratives, lending an air of credibility to their lobbying campaigns. This data-driven approach allows the industry to position itself as a knowledgeable and indispensable partner in the policymaking process, even as it seeks to influence outcomes in its favor.

Campaign contributions are another cornerstone of the insurance industry's influence. By donating to political candidates and parties across the ideological spectrum, insurers ensure access to decision-makers regardless of which party is in power. These contributions often come with implicit expectations of favorable treatment, whether in the form of supportive legislation, lenient regulatory enforcement, or opposition to proposals that threaten industry profitability. The result is a political environment in which the voices of insurers are amplified, often drowning out those of consumers, patients, and public health advocates.

The insurance industry's strategic maneuvers are not without consequences for the broader healthcare system. While insurers play a legitimate role in managing risk and facilitating access to care, their profit-driven priorities often create misalignments with the goals of affordability, equity, and quality. For example, the industry's emphasis on cost containment frequently results in practices like narrow networks, high deductibles, and prior authorization requirements, which can limit patients' access to necessary care. Additionally, the industry's lobbying efforts have often stymied attempts to introduce systemic reforms, such as single-payer models or public options, that could disrupt the status quo.

Critics argue that the insurance industry's influence perpetuates a fragmented and inefficient healthcare system that prioritizes financial gain over patient welfare. By focusing on short-term profitability, insurers may resist innovations or reforms that could lead to long-term improvements in health outcomes and cost efficiency. Furthermore, the industry's strategic maneuvers often exacerbate existing inequities, as marginalized populations are disproportionately affected by practices that limit access to care or impose financial burdens.

Despite these challenges, the insurance industry's power shows no signs of waning. As healthcare costs continue to rise and the system becomes increasingly complex, insurers remain well-positioned to shape the future of healthcare policy in the United States. Their ability to navigate the political and regulatory landscape with precision ensures that their interests will continue to be prioritized, even as calls for reform grow louder. Understanding the strategic maneuvers of the insurance industry is essential for anyone seeking to grapple with the complexities of the healthcare system and envision a path toward a more equitable and effective model of care.

BIG PHARMA: LOBBYING FOR PROFIT AND PROTECTION

The pharmaceutical industry, colloquially referred to as Big Pharma, wields a formidable influence in the American healthcare system, shaping policy decisions and regulatory frameworks to protect its profit margins and secure its dominant position. With substantial financial resources at its disposal, the industry has established itself as a lobbying powerhouse, effectively aligning government action with its commercial interests. This influence extends far beyond the halls of Congress, permeating agencies, regulatory bodies, and even public opinion.

At the core of Big Pharma's lobbying efforts lies a dual agenda: securing market exclusivity and ensuring favorable pricing mechanisms. Patent protections and regulatory exclusivities, such as those provided under the Hatch-Waxman Act and the Orphan Drug Act, serve as critical pillars of the industry's business model. Pharmaceutical companies invest heavily in lobbying to maintain and expand these protections, often under the guise of promoting innovation. They argue that extended periods of market exclusivity are essential to recoup the significant costs associated with drug research and development. While this rationale carries some validity, the industry's aggressive pursuit of these protections often results in practices that hinder competition and inflate drug prices.

The interplay between innovation and profit-seeking is exemplified in the strategies companies employ to extend patent lifespans. Practices like "evergreening," where minor modifications to existing drugs are patented as new innovations, allow companies to delay the entry of generic competitors. Lobbyists for the pharmaceutical industry have been instrumental in preserving the legal and regulatory frameworks that enable these tactics, often framing them as necessary incentives for continued investment in groundbreaking therapies. However, these strategies frequently come at a significant cost to consumers, who face inflated prices for medications long after their initial patents have expired.

In addition to protecting patents, Big Pharma exerts considerable influence over drug pricing policies. The United States remains one of the few developed nations where pharmaceutical companies can set drug prices with minimal government intervention. Lobbying efforts have played a key role in maintaining this status quo, blocking legislative attempts to introduce price controls or empower Medicare to negotiate drug prices directly. This lack of regulation has contributed to the United States having some of the highest drug prices globally, a fact often justified by the industry as a trade-off for its role as a global leader in pharmaceutical innovation.

Big Pharma's influence is not confined to federal policy but extends to state governments, where decisions about Medicaid formularies, drug pricing transparency laws, and opioid regulations are often made. Pharmaceutical companies deploy extensive lobbying resources at the state level, shaping policies that align with their interests. This localized lobbying ensures that the industry's priorities are addressed across the diverse regulatory landscapes of individual states, further entrenching its power.

Campaign donations represent another critical tool in Big Pharma's arsenal. Pharmaceutical companies and their trade organizations, such as the Pharmaceutical Research and Manufacturers of America (PhRMA), contribute millions of dollars to political candidates and parties, ensuring access and influence regardless of the prevailing political climate. These contributions are often accompanied by extensive lobbying efforts to build relationships with lawmakers, positioning the industry as a trusted partner in addressing healthcare challenges. The result is a political environment where the voices of pharmaceutical companies are amplified, often overshadowing those advocating for consumer protections or systemic reforms.

Regulatory capture is another hallmark of Big Pharma's influence. The revolving door between the pharmaceutical industry and government agencies, such as the Food and Drug Administration (FDA), creates a symbiotic relationship that often blurs the line between regulation and advocacy. Former industry executives frequently occupy key positions within regulatory bodies, while former regulators transition into lucrative roles within the industry. This dynamic fosters a regulatory environment that is often perceived as being overly accommodating to the industry's interests, raising concerns about the impartiality of oversight and the prioritization of public health.

The opioid epidemic provides a stark example of the consequences of Big Pharma's lobbying influence. For years, pharmaceutical companies downplayed the addictive potential of opioid medications while aggressively marketing them to healthcare providers. Lobbying efforts targeted lawmakers and regulators to ensure lenient policies regarding opioid prescribing and distribution. Even as the devastating consequences of opioid misuse became apparent, the industry worked to deflect responsibility and resist stricter regulations. The result was a public health crisis that underscored the dangers of prioritizing corporate interests over community well-being.

Critics of Big Pharma's lobbying practices argue that they contribute to systemic inequities within the healthcare system. By prioritizing profit over accessibility, the industry often leaves vulnerable populations without affordable access to essential medications. Moreover, the focus on high-margin drugs, such as specialty and biologic therapies, frequently comes at the expense of investments in treatments for less profitable conditions, such as rare diseases or tropical illnesses. This misalignment of priorities highlights the broader societal implications of a healthcare system heavily influenced by corporate lobbying.

Despite these criticisms, Big Pharma continues to defend its practices by emphasizing its role in advancing medical innovation. The industry points to the development of life-saving therapies, such as vaccines and cancer treatments, as evidence of its indispensable contribution to global health. While these achievements are undeniably significant, they often come with a hefty price tag, raising questions about the balance between rewarding innovation and ensuring affordability.

Addressing the influence of Big Pharma on the healthcare system requires a multifaceted approach. Policy reforms that promote transparency in drug pricing, curtail anti-competitive practices, and empower public agencies to negotiate prices could help realign the system with the goals of equity and accessibility. Additionally, efforts to strengthen regulatory oversight and mitigate the impact of the revolving door between the industry and government agencies could enhance the integrity of the policymaking process.

Ultimately, the challenge lies in balancing the legitimate needs of the pharmaceutical industry to sustain innovation with the broader societal imperative to provide affordable and equitable access to healthcare. Achieving this balance will require a concerted effort to reduce the outsized influence of Big Pharma's lobbying while fostering a healthcare system that prioritizes the well-being of patients over corporate profits.

Hospital Systems and Their Advocacy

Hospital systems occupy a unique and powerful position within the healthcare ecosystem, functioning as both providers of essential care and influential players in the political arena. As the central hubs of care delivery, hospitals wield considerable economic, social, and political influence, which they use to advocate for policies that align with their interests. While their lobbying efforts often emphasize the challenges of delivering quality care in a complex and underfunded system, they also reveal the financial and competitive motivations driving hospital systems to secure their dominant positions.

The advocacy efforts of hospital systems are deeply tied to their dual roles as public health institutions and significant economic entities. On the one hand, hospitals frame their lobbying initiatives around the need to maintain access to care, particularly for vulnerable populations. This is especially true for nonprofit hospitals, which often highlight their community benefit obligations and reliance on government programs like Medicare and Medicaid to support their mission. These hospitals frequently advocate for increased funding for these programs, arguing that cuts would jeopardize their ability to serve underserved populations. On the surface, this aligns with public health priorities, but it also underscores the financial dependence of hospitals on government reimbursement mechanisms.

However, the distinction between nonprofit and for-profit hospitals often blurs when examining lobbying strategies, as both types of institutions are deeply invested in shaping policies that ensure financial stability and growth. For example, hospital systems have been staunch opponents of efforts to expand site-neutral payment policies, which aim to standardize reimbursement rates for similar services regardless of where they are delivered. Hospitals argue that these policies fail to account for the higher costs associated with operating comprehensive care facilities. Critics, however, suggest that opposition to site-neutral payments is driven more by the desire to protect lucrative revenue streams than by a commitment to care delivery.

Another key area of hospital advocacy centers on issues of consolidation and market power. Over the past few decades, the healthcare landscape has witnessed a significant wave of hospital mergers and acquisitions, resulting in the formation of large health systems with considerable market influence. These consolidated systems argue that integration enhances efficiency, improves patient outcomes, and reduces costs by leveraging economies of scale. While there is some evidence to support these claims, the broader impact of consolidation has been mixed. In many cases, hospital mergers have led to higher prices for consumers and insurers, as consolidated systems use their market power to negotiate more favorable reimbursement rates. Lobbying efforts in this context often aim to counter regulatory scrutiny and antitrust actions, framing consolidation as a necessary response to economic pressures rather than a strategy to dominate regional markets.

The influence of hospital systems extends to federal and state legislatures, where they advocate for policies that protect their interests. Campaign contributions from hospital-affiliated political action committees (PACs) and trade organizations such as the American Hospital Association (AHA) play a significant role in shaping legislative priorities. These contributions are often directed toward lawmakers with jurisdiction over health policy, ensuring that hospital perspectives are well-represented in debates over reimbursement rates, funding allocations, and regulatory frameworks. At the same time, hospital systems invest heavily in direct lobbying efforts, employing teams of experts to engage with policymakers and provide data that supports their positions.

One of the most contentious areas of hospital advocacy is the issue of surprise billing, which occurs when patients receive unexpected charges for out-of-network care during emergencies or hospital visits. Hospitals have frequently been at the center of this debate, as they negotiate contracts with insurers that determine which providers are considered in-network. While hospitals often blame insurers for inadequate network coverage, their lobbying efforts have at times resisted comprehensive reforms that would eliminate surprise billing altogether. Instead, they have advocated for arbitration mechanisms that allow them to resolve disputes with insurers on terms favorable to their financial interests. These positions highlight the tension between hospitals' public health narratives and their financial motivations, particularly when patient interests are caught in the crossfire.

The role of hospitals in Medicaid expansion debates further illustrates their complex advocacy strategies. In states where Medicaid expansion under the Affordable Care Act has been politically contentious, hospitals have been among the most vocal proponents of expansion. They argue that extending Medicaid coverage to more low-income individuals reduces the burden of uncompensated care and improves financial stability for hospitals serving large numbers of uninsured patients. While this advocacy aligns with broader public health goals, it also reflects the financial realities facing hospitals, which must navigate thin margins and increasing competition in a challenging economic environment.

Despite their significant resources and influence, hospital systems face growing scrutiny over their financial practices and lobbying priorities. Critics argue that hospitals often prioritize revenue generation over patient care, pointing to instances where high charges, aggressive debt collection practices, and opaque billing systems undermine their public health missions. For nonprofit hospitals, these criticisms are particularly pointed, as their tax-exempt status is contingent on demonstrating substantial community benefits. Advocacy efforts in this context often aim to counter negative perceptions, emphasizing the role of hospitals as safety nets and essential providers.

Addressing the influence of hospital advocacy requires a nuanced approach that recognizes both their essential contributions to healthcare and the financial motivations that drive their lobbying efforts. Policymakers and regulators must strike a balance between supporting hospitals' ability to deliver high-quality care and ensuring that their actions align with the broader goals of affordability, equity, and transparency. Greater oversight of hospital consolidation, pricing practices, and lobbying activities could help mitigate some of the negative impacts of their influence while preserving their vital role in the healthcare system.

Ultimately, hospital systems embody the complexities of the American healthcare system, where the imperatives of public service and financial sustainability are inextricably linked. Their advocacy efforts, while often framed as efforts to protect access and quality, reveal the underlying economic pressures and competitive dynamics that shape their priorities. Understanding and addressing these dynamics is essential for creating a healthcare system that truly serves the needs of patients and communities.

Campaign Financing: Buying Influence, Shaping Policy

The intricate web of campaign financing reveals how financial contributions from powerful healthcare entities subtly, yet profoundly, shape the political landscape. In the United States, campaign donations have become an essential tool for industries seeking to influence policymakers, and healthcare is no exception. At the heart of this dynamic lies a tacit exchange: financial support for elected officials in return for legislative and regulatory decisions that align with the interests of donors. The vast resources funneled into political campaigns by the insurance, pharmaceutical, and hospital industries exemplify this exchange, revealing the profound impact of money on healthcare policy.

Campaign financing begins with the political action committees (PACs) established by major players in the healthcare sector. These committees function as conduits through which corporate funds flow into the coffers of candidates who support industry-friendly policies. The sheer scale of these contributions is staggering, with millions of dollars donated during each election cycle. Insurers, pharmaceutical companies, and hospital systems are among the largest contributors, each vying for influence over the legislators and executives who determine the rules of the game. The recipients of these funds are carefully chosen, often including members of key congressional committees tasked with overseeing health policy and appropriations.

The power of campaign donations is most evident in the legislative outcomes that follow. Lawmakers who receive significant contributions from the healthcare industry often become champions of policies that protect and enhance the profitability of their benefactors. For instance, pharmaceutical companies have long leveraged campaign financing to resist efforts to regulate drug prices. By directing funds to candidates who oppose price controls, the industry has successfully delayed or watered down legislation that threatens its profit margins. Similarly, the insurance industry has used campaign donations to influence debates over coverage mandates and consumer protections, ensuring that reforms do not compromise their bottom lines.

The influence of campaign financing extends beyond direct legislative action to the broader regulatory environment. Industries that invest heavily in campaign contributions often enjoy privileged access to policymakers, allowing them to shape the implementation of laws and regulations. This access manifests in meetings, hearings, and advisory roles where industry representatives present their perspectives as stakeholders. Such influence can result in regulations that reflect the priorities of donors rather than the public interest, perpetuating a cycle of policy-making that favors corporate interests.

Campaign financing also plays a critical role in shaping public opinion and electoral outcomes. The funds provided by healthcare PACs are often used to support advertising campaigns, voter outreach efforts, and other activities that bolster the electoral prospects of favored candidates. These activities, while ostensibly separate from direct lobbying, serve to amplify the voices of industry-aligned policymakers and marginalize dissenting perspectives. The result is an electoral landscape where candidates who challenge the status quo face significant financial disadvantages, reducing the likelihood of transformative reforms.

While campaign contributions are legal and subject to disclosure requirements, the opacity of certain funding mechanisms complicates efforts to trace the influence of money in politics. Super PACs and dark money organizations, which can accept unlimited contributions and are not required to disclose their donors, further obscure the relationship between campaign financing and policy outcomes. These entities allow healthcare corporations to wield influence indirectly, funding advertisements and advocacy campaigns that shape the narrative around key issues without overtly tying the messaging to corporate interests.

The interplay between campaign financing and healthcare policy raises fundamental questions about democratic accountability. When industries with vested financial interests dominate political donations, the risk of policy capture becomes pronounced. This phenomenon occurs when policymakers prioritize the preferences of donors over the needs of constituents, undermining the principles of representative democracy. In the context of healthcare, the consequences of policy capture are particularly severe, as decisions influenced by corporate contributions can have profound implications for access, affordability, and quality of care.

Addressing the influence of campaign financing on healthcare policy requires comprehensive reform. Efforts to limit the size of individual contributions, increase transparency in donor reporting, and restrict the activities of dark money organizations are essential steps toward reducing the outsized influence of corporate interests. Public financing of campaigns, which provides candidates with funding independent of private donations, offers another promising avenue for leveling the playing field and ensuring that policymakers are accountable to their constituents rather than their donors.

Yet, the path to reform is fraught with challenges, not least because the very system that perpetuates corporate influence also empowers those who would resist change. The entrenched interests benefiting from the status quo are unlikely to support measures that curtail their power, necessitating grassroots mobilization and public pressure to drive reform. Advocacy organizations, citizen groups, and independent media have a critical role to play in exposing the connections between campaign financing and policy outcomes, fostering greater awareness and demand for accountability.

The pervasive influence of campaign financing on healthcare policy underscores the need for vigilance and action to safeguard the integrity of democratic processes. As long as the flow of money into politics remains unchecked, the healthcare system will continue to reflect the priorities of its most powerful stakeholders rather than the needs of the people it serves. Breaking this cycle is essential for creating a more equitable and responsive healthcare system, one where policies are guided by the principles of public health and social justice rather than the dictates of corporate profit.

Corporate Interests Versus Public Health

The tension between corporate interests and public health lies at the heart of the healthcare debate, exposing the inherent conflicts that arise when profit-driven entities exert significant influence over a system designed to prioritize human well-being. This dynamic is not unique to the United States but is particularly pronounced within its highly privatized healthcare structure, where corporations often dictate the terms of access, pricing, and care delivery. The consequences of this imbalance are profound, manifesting in policies and practices that frequently prioritize shareholder returns over equitable health outcomes.

At the very center, the conflict stems from divergent priorities. Public health emphasizes the collective well-being of communities, striving for universal access to preventative care, affordable treatments, and robust disease management systems. Corporate entities in healthcare, by contrast, operate within a framework that prioritizes financial growth and competitive advantage. These opposing objectives create a fundamental misalignment that shapes the healthcare landscape in ways that often exacerbate disparities and limit systemic progress.

The pharmaceutical industry exemplifies this clash. While innovation in drug development is undeniably crucial for advancing medical science, the profit motives driving pharmaceutical corporations can lead to pricing strategies that make life-saving medications inaccessible to large segments of the population. The astronomical costs of certain treatments, such as those for rare diseases or cutting-edge oncology therapies, reflect not only the expenses of research and development but also the market-driven imperatives of maximizing returns. These prices force patients, insurers, and government programs to bear enormous financial burdens, often at the expense of broader public health initiatives.

Corporate interests also significantly shape the insurance industry, where the business model inherently depends on balancing risk and profitability. This creates incentives to limit coverage, exclude high-risk patients, or increase premiums, particularly in the absence of robust regulatory oversight. The resulting gaps in access leave millions of individuals either uninsured or underinsured, unable to obtain necessary care. This dynamic disproportionately impacts vulnerable populations, further entrenching health inequities and undermining the foundational goals of public health.

Hospital systems, increasingly dominated by large corporate entities, also illustrate the tension between profitability and care quality. The consolidation of healthcare facilities into vast networks has created regional monopolies that can dictate pricing and prioritize high-margin services, such as elective procedures, over essential but less profitable care areas like mental health or primary care. These trends contribute to rising healthcare costs and create geographic disparities, where rural or underserved areas struggle to maintain basic medical infrastructure.

One of the most insidious effects of corporate dominance in healthcare is its impact on policy-making. Through lobbying, campaign donations, and other forms of influence, healthcare corporations shape the legislative and regulatory frameworks that govern the system. This often results in policies that protect corporate interests at the expense of public health. For example, intellectual property laws designed to encourage innovation have also been exploited to extend patent protections and delay the entry of more affordable generic drugs into the market. Similarly, resistance to price transparency measures and aggressive lobbying against universal healthcare proposals reflect the industry's prioritization of profits over systemic reform.

The effects of corporate influence extend beyond economic barriers to care, seeping into the realm of public trust. When patients perceive that their health is commodified—that decisions about their care are driven more by financial interests than medical necessity—confidence in the system erodes. This distrust has significant implications, including reduced adherence to medical advice, increased reliance on alternative and often unproven therapies, and a growing skepticism toward public health campaigns. The COVID-19 pandemic underscored this dynamic, with debates over vaccine access and pricing further highlighting the clash between public health imperatives and corporate profit motives.

Despite these challenges, the relationship between corporate interests and public health is not uniformly antagonistic. Many corporations have made significant contributions to advancing medical science, expanding access to care, and addressing pressing public health needs. Pharmaceutical companies, for instance, were pivotal in developing COVID-19 vaccines in record time, leveraging resources and expertise to combat a global crisis. Similarly, hospital systems have innovated in care delivery models, integrating technology and data analytics to improve patient outcomes. These examples demonstrate that aligning corporate success with public health goals is not only possible but also necessary for achieving sustainable improvements in the healthcare system.

Addressing the conflict between corporate interests and public health requires a multifaceted approach. Policymakers must implement stronger regulatory frameworks to ensure that profitability does not come at the expense of accessibility or equity. This includes measures such as capping drug prices, mandating coverage of essential health services, and incentivizing investments in underserved communities. Transparency is also critical, with robust reporting requirements for pricing, lobbying activities, and corporate financial practices to hold healthcare entities accountable.

Public engagement is another essential component of realigning the system. Grassroots movements, advocacy groups, and consumer organizations have the power to challenge corporate practices that undermine public health. By demanding accountability and pushing for systemic reforms, these groups can counterbalance the influence of corporate lobbying and ensure that the voices of patients and communities are heard in policy debates.

Ultimately, the interplay between corporate interests and public health reflects broader societal choices about the values that should underpin the healthcare system. Striking a balance between innovation and accessibility, profitability and equity, requires a commitment to placing human well-being at the center of the system. This vision demands not only policy changes but also a cultural shift that prioritizes collaboration over competition, compassion over commodification, and the collective good over individual gain. Only by addressing these underlying tensions can the healthcare system evolve to meet the needs of all, rather than serving the interests of a privileged few.

Balancing Power: Counter-Lobbying and Grassroots Movements

Amid the outsized influence of healthcare lobbying, grassroots movements and counter-lobbying efforts have emerged as powerful forces challenging the status quo. These groups aim to shift the balance of power away from corporate interests and towards policies that prioritize accessibility, equity, and the public good. The rise of such movements highlights the growing awareness among citizens, patient advocates, and reform-minded policymakers that unchecked corporate influence not only undermines public trust but also perpetuates a healthcare system that often fails its most vulnerable members.

Grassroots movements in healthcare are typically driven by personal stories of struggle, injustice, and financial hardship. Families bankrupt by medical bills, patients denied life-saving treatments due to insurer loopholes, and communities devastated by hospital closures have all become rallying points for collective action. These movements use the emotional weight of these stories to generate public sympathy, galvanize support, and exert pressure on policymakers to address systemic inequities. Unlike corporate lobbyists, whose power lies in financial resources, grassroots organizations draw strength from their ability to mobilize public opinion and amplify the voices of ordinary citizens.

One of the most notable examples of grassroots healthcare advocacy in recent history is the campaign to protect the Affordable Care Act (ACA) from repeal efforts. When legislative attempts to dismantle the ACA gained traction, a diverse coalition of patients, healthcare workers, and community leaders organized rallies, town hall meetings, and social media campaigns to underscore the potential human cost of losing access to care. These efforts played a critical role in swaying public opinion and influencing key votes, demonstrating the capacity of grassroots advocacy to counter even the most well-funded lobbying campaigns.

Grassroots movements also serve as a counterbalance to corporate lobbying by focusing on transparency and accountability. Organizations such as Public Citizen and Patients for Affordable Drugs have made it their mission to expose the financial ties between lawmakers and the healthcare industry, shedding light on the ways in which campaign contributions and lobbying expenditures shape policy outcomes. By making this information publicly accessible, these groups empower voters to hold elected officials accountable for decisions that prioritize corporate interests over public health.

Counter-lobbying efforts have also emerged within professional healthcare organizations and unions. Physicians, nurses, and other healthcare workers have increasingly organized to advocate for policies that align with their ethical commitment to patient care. For instance, groups like Physicians for a National Health Program (PNHP) have been vocal proponents of single-payer healthcare, arguing that such a system would reduce administrative burdens, lower costs, and improve outcomes. These professionals bring credibility and expertise to the debate, countering the often profit-driven narratives advanced by corporate stakeholders.

Technology and social media have further amplified the impact of grassroots movements. Digital platforms allow advocates to disseminate information, organize campaigns, and mobilize supporters on an unprecedented scale. Hashtags like #MedicareForAll and #PatientsOverProfits have become rallying cries for reform, uniting disparate groups under a common cause. The viral nature of social media campaigns enables these movements to reach a broad audience, generating momentum that can translate into tangible policy changes.

Despite their successes, grassroots movements face significant challenges in countering the entrenched power of healthcare corporations. Financial disparities between grassroots organizations and industry lobbyists remain stark, limiting the former's ability to compete in terms of access to policymakers and media visibility. Moreover, the decentralized nature of grassroots advocacy can make it difficult to sustain momentum and achieve cohesion around specific policy goals. Fragmentation within these movements—whether over ideological differences or strategic approaches—can dilute their impact and make them vulnerable to co-optation by more powerful interests.

The role of unions and professional organizations in counter-lobbying also highlights an important dynamic: while these groups advocate for systemic reforms, they often face internal conflicts of interest. For example, unions representing healthcare workers may push for policies that benefit their members, such as higher wages or better working conditions, even if these priorities occasionally conflict with broader public health goals. Navigating these complexities requires a careful balance between advancing the interests of specific constituencies and promoting systemic equity.

Despite these obstacles, the potential of grassroots and counter-lobbying efforts to drive meaningful change in healthcare policy cannot be overstated. These movements remind us that the power of collective action, when strategically harnessed, can challenge even the most entrenched systems. They also underscore the importance of democracy in policymaking, ensuring that the voices of patients, caregivers, and communities are not drowned out by corporate interests.

To enhance their impact, grassroots movements must continue to build alliances across sectors and demographics, uniting diverse stakeholders under a shared vision of a fairer and more equitable healthcare system. Leveraging data, storytelling, and innovative advocacy strategies can help these groups maintain momentum and expand their influence. Additionally, fostering partnerships with reform-minded policymakers and philanthropic organizations can provide the resources and institutional support needed to sustain their efforts.

Ultimately, the struggle to balance corporate power with grassroots advocacy is not just a battle over healthcare policy; it is a broader fight for social justice and democratic accountability. By challenging the dominance of profit-driven interests, these movements aim to create a healthcare system that reflects our collective values—one that prioritizes compassion, accessibility, and equity over financial gain. This vision, while ambitious, is essential for building a future where healthcare is not a privilege reserved for the few but a fundamental right for all.

Looking Forward: Reforming the Lobbying Ecosystem

Reforming the lobbying ecosystem within the healthcare sector demands a multifaceted approach that balances the legitimate role of advocacy with the need to prioritize public health over private profit. Lobbying, in its ideal form, is a mechanism through which various stakeholders can voice their perspectives, contribute expertise, and shape policy in ways that reflect the complexities of the healthcare landscape. Yet, in its current state, the system disproportionately serves the interests of those with the deepest pockets, perpetuating inequities and undermining trust in both the industry and government. Moving forward, creating a lobbying framework that emphasizes accountability, transparency, and equity will be critical to aligning healthcare policy with the broader public interest.

At the heart of lobbying reform is the need for greater transparency. One of the most effective steps toward this goal is mandating full disclosure of lobbying activities, including the amounts spent, the policies targeted, and the specific interactions between lobbyists and lawmakers. Enhanced reporting requirements would allow journalists, watchdog organizations, and the public to scrutinize the influence exerted by corporations on healthcare legislation. Digital tools could play a crucial role here, enabling real-time tracking of lobbying expenditures and their connections to policy outcomes. Such transparency would not only foster accountability but also help rebuild public trust in the legislative process.

Another critical area for reform is campaign finance. The intimate relationship between lobbying expenditures and political campaign contributions creates an environment where policy decisions often reflect donor priorities rather than public needs. Introducing stricter limits on campaign donations from healthcare entities—especially those with direct financial stakes in the outcomes—could help mitigate this imbalance. Public financing of political campaigns is another potential solution, reducing candidates' reliance on corporate contributions and leveling the playing field for reform-minded leaders who lack the backing of major industry players.

To counteract the outsized influence of corporate lobbyists, it is essential to amplify the voices of other stakeholders, including patients, healthcare workers, and public health advocates. Establishing dedicated avenues for these groups to participate in the policymaking process—such as citizen advisory boards, public hearings, or grassroots advocacy grants—can provide a counterbalance to the dominance of industry interests. Ensuring that these voices are not merely heard but actively incorporated into legislative deliberations would signal a commitment to democratic decision-making and equity in healthcare reform.

Regulating the revolving door between industry and government is another essential component of reform. The frequent exchange of personnel between these two spheres creates significant conflicts of interest, as policymakers with industry ties may prioritize corporate agendas over public welfare. Imposing stricter cooling-off periods—requiring former government officials to wait several years before joining lobbying firms or corporate boards—would reduce the potential for undue influence. Similarly, implementing robust conflict-of-interest laws could help ensure that individuals in key policymaking positions act in the public's best interest rather than advancing private-sector goals.

Reforming the lobbying ecosystem also necessitates addressing the systemic disparities that make grassroots and counter-lobbying efforts inherently disadvantaged. Providing public funding or tax incentives for nonprofit advocacy groups focused on healthcare equity could help level the playing field, allowing these organizations to compete more effectively with corporate interests. Encouraging philanthropic foundations to support policy advocacy work in the healthcare sector is another strategy for bolstering the resources available to reform-oriented movements.

International models can provide valuable lessons for reforming the U.S. lobbying landscape. In countries where healthcare systems are more centralized, such as the United Kingdom or Canada, the influence of industry lobbying is often more constrained due to stronger regulations and a greater emphasis on public accountability. Adapting elements of these systems—such as independent commissions to oversee lobbying practices—could help address some of the most egregious abuses of power within the U.S. context while respecting the unique dynamics of its healthcare system.

While these reforms present viable pathways for change, the entrenched power of the healthcare lobby means that achieving meaningful transformation will require sustained effort and political will. It is not enough to pass individual pieces of legislation; systemic change demands a cultural shift in how healthcare is viewed and prioritized within the political arena. Policymakers must recognize that the health of their constituents is not merely a budgetary concern or an economic driver but a fundamental determinant of societal well-being and cohesion.

Public engagement is key to driving this cultural shift. Educating citizens about the role of lobbying in shaping their healthcare system—and empowering them to demand greater accountability—can create the political pressure necessary for reform. Movements that successfully mobilize public opinion, such as those advocating for drug price reductions or universal healthcare, demonstrate the potential of collective action to challenge the dominance of corporate interests. These movements must be sustained and expanded, drawing in diverse coalitions that transcend partisan divides and focus on shared goals.

Reforming the lobbying ecosystem is not just about limiting the influence of corporate power; it is about reimagining the role of advocacy in a way that prioritizes the health and well-being of all Americans. By creating a system that values transparency, equity, and democratic participation, it is possible to build a healthcare landscape that reflects the needs and aspirations of the people it serves. Such a transformation will not happen overnight, but with persistent effort and a commitment to justice, it is a vision well within reach.

Chapter 9: Reform or Rhetoric? The Cycles of Healthcare Debate

The United States is a country built on paradoxes, and its healthcare debate is no exception. On one hand, polls consistently reveal widespread public dissatisfaction with the current system: Americans routinely identify healthcare reform as a pressing national priority. On the other hand, when it comes to specific proposals, this apparent consensus shatters into fragmented interests, ideological divides, and unbridgeable partisan gaps. The healthcare debate is, at its core, a cyclical struggle between collective aspiration and deeply entrenched resistance—a pattern that raises the question: why does consensus so often prove to be a mirage?

At the surface, it seems simple. Americans overwhelmingly agree on the broad strokes: healthcare costs too much, leaves too many uninsured or underinsured, and too often prioritizes profit over patient care. The data supports this frustration. The United States spends more per capita on healthcare than any other nation, yet millions remain without access to adequate care. Metrics of health outcomes, such as life expectancy and maternal mortality, frequently lag behind those of other developed countries. By these standards, there is every reason to expect that a unified public would demand bold, transformative solutions. But the history of healthcare reform tells a different story, one of cyclical debates that fizzle into compromises, rhetorical stalemates, or outright abandonment of sweeping proposals.

This cycle begins with what appears to be national momentum. Crises in the system—escalating costs, shocking statistics, or high-profile tragedies—trigger waves of public outcry. Politicians seize the moment, introducing ambitious reform plans promising to fix what is broken. Yet, as the debate progresses, the initial consensus unravels. The public sphere becomes saturated with competing narratives, and reforms that once seemed urgent morph into polarizing battlegrounds. Stakeholders, from lobbyists to media pundits, flood the conversation with misinformation, fear-mongering, and appeals to self-interest. Suddenly, the lines of agreement become blurred, and the public's energy dissipates into doubt and division.

This phenomenon, the myth of consensus, is rooted in the unique cultural and ideological fabric of the United States. Americans are not merely grappling with the mechanics of healthcare reform; they are navigating a deeper clash of values. The concept of healthcare as a universal right, foundational in many

European systems, conflicts with the American ethos of individual responsibility and distrust of centralized authority. Reform efforts must contend not just with logistical and financial obstacles but with the cultural weight of a society that prizes autonomy over collectivism and competition over solidarity.

What makes this myth of consensus so enduring is that it operates on multiple levels. On the political front, bipartisan agreement on healthcare is rare, and reform efforts inevitably fall victim to gridlock. Even when the majority of the electorate supports policies like expanding Medicare or capping drug prices, partisan dynamics convert majority will into legislative paralysis. Economically, the entrenched power of the healthcare industry acts as a formidable counterweight to reform, ensuring that transformative proposals never gain sufficient traction. Culturally, the public itself becomes a fractured entity, as Americans' attitudes toward reform are shaped not just by facts but by narratives of fear, freedom, and identity.

The enduring myth of consensus also thrives on the rhetorical tactics of reform opponents. Proposals for universal healthcare, for example, are labeled as "socialist experiments" destined to collapse under bureaucratic inefficiency. Conversely, incremental changes are dismissed as Band-Aids on a hemorrhaging wound. These arguments, while often baseless, are effective in sowing doubt. They resonate with deeper anxieties about government control, economic disruption, and personal choice, ensuring that public agreement dissolves as soon as the complexities of reform are unpacked.

The myth of consensus is, perhaps, not a failure of the public's will but a testament to the systemic forces arrayed against it. Reform debates do not take place in a vacuum; they are conducted in an environment shaped by powerful interests, cultural divisions, and a political system that rewards caution over courage. In this sense, the healthcare debate in the United States is less about solving problems than it is about managing expectations—about giving the appearance of progress while leaving the underlying structures intact.

As the stage is set for each new reform effort, the same cycle repeats itself. The public calls for change, but consensus, as a vehicle for meaningful transformation, remains elusive. Instead, it becomes a rhetorical tool—invoked to galvanize support but abandoned when the details are debated. The illusion of consensus is powerful, but it is also fragile, easily shattered by the forces of ideology, politics, and economics that define the American experience.

To understand why healthcare reform remains such an intractable challenge, one must begin here: with the recognition that consensus, though seemingly within reach, is an illusion carefully maintained by the system itself. What appears to be unity is, in fact, a fault line—a reflection of the contradictions that lie at the heart of America's approach to healthcare and, perhaps, to governance as a whole.

The Anatomy of Reform Failure

Reform in the American healthcare system has long been a Sisyphean endeavor. Bold ideas, even when they gain traction, consistently falter under the weight of political inertia, economic interests, and cultural resistance. The anatomy of reform failure in the United States is a dissection of both systemic dysfunction and deliberate obstruction—a pattern that reveals not just why sweeping changes fail but why the system continues to resist even the most incremental progress.

At the heart of this persistent failure lies a fundamental contradiction: the healthcare system, designed to serve as a public good, is deeply embedded in the machinery of capitalism. Unlike in many other developed nations, where healthcare reform operates within a predominantly public framework, the American system is beholden to private interests. From pharmaceutical companies to insurance providers, hospitals to medical device manufacturers, the industry's stakeholders are structured not around the principles of universal care but around profit maximization. This profit-driven architecture creates a significant obstacle to reform, as any proposal for systemic change inherently threatens the financial incentives of some of the most powerful players in the economy.

The failure of reform, however, cannot be attributed solely to economic interests. It is equally rooted in the political machinery of the United States, which rewards incrementalism and punishes bold action. The very structure of American governance—with its checks and balances, fragmented power centers, and deep-seated partisanship—renders sweeping reforms extraordinarily difficult to achieve. Even when political will exists, it is often thwarted by the realities of legislative compromise. Ambitious proposals become diluted in the pursuit of bipartisan support, leaving reform efforts watered down and ineffective. The result is a vicious cycle: watered-down reforms fail to deliver meaningful change, further eroding public trust in the possibility of transformative solutions.

Cultural resistance compounds these structural barriers. The United States is unique in its deeply ingrained suspicion of government intervention. Proposals for universal healthcare, for example, are often met with accusations of "socialism"—a label that taps into centuries of American individualism and the fear of centralized control. This cultural skepticism extends beyond partisan lines, shaping public attitudes toward reform in ways that transcend traditional political divides. The idea of healthcare as a collective right, foundational in other nations, struggles to gain traction in a society where autonomy and self-reliance are lionized.

The anatomy of reform failure is also characterized by the role of strategic misinformation. Lobbyists and interest groups opposing reform exploit this cultural skepticism to great effect, deploying fear-based messaging to erode public support for change. The infamous "death panels" rhetoric during the Affordable Care Act debates, for instance, was a masterclass in disinformation. Such narratives play into existing anxieties about loss of choice and government overreach, ensuring that even well-intentioned reforms are viewed with suspicion. The power of these narratives lies in their simplicity—they reduce complex policy debates into emotional appeals, making them far more resonant than the intricate arguments of reform advocates.

Even when reforms manage to overcome these obstacles, they often fail in implementation. The compromises made to pass legislation frequently result in systems too convoluted or underfunded to achieve their intended goals. The Affordable Care Act, for instance, expanded access to insurance but left millions uninsured due to political concessions that excluded a public option. The failure to address underlying cost structures—such as skyrocketing drug prices and administrative overhead—meant that many Americans experienced little relief, fueling disillusionment with the reforms themselves.

The anatomy of reform failure also includes the cyclical nature of healthcare debates. Every new administration brings a fresh round of proposals, each heralded as the solution to a broken system. Yet these cycles rarely move the needle. Instead, they perpetuate a narrative of near-reform: the idea that meaningful change is always on the horizon, just out of reach. This narrative serves a dual purpose. It placates public demands for action while ensuring that the system's foundational structure remains largely intact. In this sense, the failure of reform is not an aberration but a feature of a system designed to resist disruption.

Perhaps the most tragic aspect of reform failure is its human cost. While policymakers argue over ideology and interest groups protect their profits, millions of Americans face the harsh realities of an inaccessible healthcare system. Families are bankrupted by medical bills, individuals forego necessary treatments due to cost, and preventable deaths occur in a nation that spends more on healthcare than any other. The disconnect between the promises of reform and the lived experiences of those the system is supposed to serve highlights the profound moral failure embedded within the anatomy of reform.

Reform in American healthcare does not fail because of a lack of ideas or public demand. It fails because the system is structured to resist change—economically, politically, and culturally. To understand why sweeping reforms remain elusive, one must look beyond the surface debates and examine the deeper forces at play. Only then can the persistent failure of reform be seen not as a temporary setback but as a reflection of a system that, by design, works precisely as intended—for those it was built to serve.

Incrementalism as the Path of Least Resistance

Incrementalism in American healthcare reform is not merely a strategy; it is a necessity born out of a system that vehemently resists sweeping changes. This piecemeal approach to reform represents the path of least resistance, where small adjustments are made to address glaring inefficiencies without challenging the system's foundational structure. It is a strategy shaped by political pragmatism, corporate influence, and cultural compromise—one that often perpetuates the very issues it seeks to resolve.

At its essence, incrementalism emerges from the impossibility of consensus in American politics. Unlike the healthcare systems of other developed nations, which often stem from a shared post-war consensus on universal care, the United States lacks a unified vision of what healthcare should look like. Instead, debates are fractured along ideological lines, with conservatives prioritizing market freedom and limited government, and progressives advocating for expanded access and government intervention. In such an environment, sweeping reforms—such as the implementation of a single-payer system—face insurmountable opposition. Incremental change, by contrast, offers a politically palatable alternative that can garner enough bipartisan support to move forward, even if only by inches.

This incrementalist ethos is vividly illustrated in the history of American healthcare reform. Landmark changes, such as the introduction of Medicare and Medicaid in 1965, were the result of decades of political negotiation and compromise. These programs, though transformative for the populations they serve, were not universal in scope. Instead, they carved out specific demographics—seniors, low-income families, and people with disabilities—while leaving the broader system intact. Subsequent reforms, from the expansion of Medicaid under the Affordable Care Act to the implementation of value-based payment models, have followed the same pattern: targeted solutions that address specific gaps without fundamentally altering the private, profit-driven nature of the healthcare system.

This reliance on incrementalism has profound consequences. While it allows for the passage of reforms that would otherwise be politically unfeasible, it also results in a patchwork system that struggles to function cohesively. Each new reform adds layers of complexity, creating a system that is increasingly difficult to navigate for both providers and patients. The result is a healthcare landscape riddled with inefficiencies, where costs continue to soar, and access remains uneven. Incrementalism, by avoiding confrontation with the system's structural flaws, often exacerbates the very problems it seeks to address.

Economically, incrementalism benefits the entrenched interests that dominate the American healthcare landscape. Pharmaceutical companies, insurance providers, and hospital systems—all of which wield immense lobbying power—have little incentive to support reforms that threaten their profit margins. Incremental changes, however, allow these stakeholders to adapt without significant disruption. They can adjust to new regulations, find loopholes, or shift costs to other parts of the system, ensuring their profitability remains intact. In this sense, incrementalism not only reflects political pragmatism but also economic preservation. It is a form of change that aligns with the interests of those who benefit most from the status quo.

Culturally, incrementalism aligns with the American ethos of individualism and limited government intervention. Sweeping reforms, such as single-payer healthcare, are often framed as an assault on personal freedom—an argument that resonates deeply in a society that prizes autonomy and choice. Incremental changes, by contrast, are seen as less intrusive. They promise improvement without fundamentally altering the relationship between individuals and the state. This cultural acceptance of incrementalism, however, comes at a cost. It reinforces the perception that transformative change is both undesirable and unachievable, further entrenching the status quo.

Even within the context of the Affordable Care Act, incrementalism's limitations are evident. The ACA, hailed as a monumental achievement in healthcare reform, was built on compromises that ultimately constrained its impact. While it expanded insurance coverage to millions of Americans, it stopped short of creating a public option or addressing the underlying cost structures of care. As a result, many of the systemic issues—skyrocketing premiums, unaffordable prescription drugs, and fragmented care delivery—remain unresolved. The ACA exemplifies how incrementalism, though politically necessary, often falls short of delivering the transformative change that advocates envision.

Despite its shortcomings, incrementalism persists because it is the only viable path forward in a deeply divided system. It represents a form of pragmatic idealism—a recognition that while sweeping reforms may be desirable, they are not achievable within the current political and economic landscape. Incrementalism offers a way to address immediate needs, even if it does so imperfectly. It provides a mechanism for progress, however slow, in a system where gridlock often prevails.

However, the reliance on incrementalism also raises critical questions about the future of healthcare reform in the United States. Can a system built on piecemeal changes ever achieve the coherence and equity seen in other nations? Or does incrementalism merely perpetuate a cycle of half-measures that fail to address the system's underlying flaws? These questions underscore the paradox of incrementalism: it is both a tool for progress and a barrier to transformative change.

In the anatomy of reform, incrementalism is the connective tissue—a strategy that binds together disparate efforts to improve the system without dismantling its foundations. It is a compromise between the ideal and the possible, the sweeping vision and the political reality. But as the healthcare debates continue to unfold, the limitations of incrementalism become increasingly apparent. The challenge lies not only in navigating the path of least resistance but in envisioning a future where the need for such resistance is finally overcome.

THE SINGLE-PAYER DEBATE—A NATION DIVIDED

The single-payer healthcare debate in the United States encapsulates the ideological, economic, and cultural divisions that define the nation's approach to reform. At its core, it represents a clash of values: collectivism versus individualism, equity versus liberty, and government intervention versus market-driven solutions. While the single-payer model has gained traction as a potential solution to the inefficiencies and inequities of the current system, it remains one of the most polarizing issues in American politics. The debate over its feasibility and desirability reflects not only divergent views on healthcare but also the broader ideological fault lines that permeate the country's political and social fabric.

Proponents of single-payer healthcare argue that it is the most effective way to achieve universal coverage, reduce administrative waste, and control rising healthcare costs. In such a system, the government assumes the role of a single insurer, streamlining the payment process and ensuring that all citizens have access to care. Advocates often point to the success of similar systems in other developed nations, such as Canada and the United Kingdom, where single-payer models have delivered higher health outcomes at lower per-capita costs. For them, the moral imperative is clear: healthcare is a human right, and a single-payer system is the most equitable and efficient way to fulfill that right.

Opponents, however, counter with concerns about the potential consequences of such a radical overhaul. Critics argue that single-payer healthcare would stifle innovation, burden taxpayers with unsustainable costs, and lead to government overreach in personal healthcare decisions. The fear of long wait times, limited provider choice, and bureaucratic inefficiencies looms large in the minds of many Americans, fueled in part by targeted campaigns from vested interests in the private sector. For these critics, the single-payer model represents not a solution but a threat—a step toward socialism that undermines the principles of free enterprise and individual autonomy.

The resistance to single-payer healthcare is not only ideological but also deeply entrenched in the political and economic structures of the United States. The private insurance industry, which generates billions of dollars in annual revenue, has a vested interest in maintaining the status quo. This industry wields considerable lobbying power, influencing legislation and shaping public perception through well-funded campaigns. Similarly, pharmaceutical companies, hospital systems, and medical device manufacturers have little incentive to support a system that might reduce their profit margins. Together, these stakeholders form a powerful coalition that actively works to stifle momentum for single-payer reform.

Culturally, the single-payer debate taps into the American ethos of self-reliance and skepticism of government intervention. Unlike many European nations, where the social contract includes a strong commitment to universal healthcare, the United States has historically prioritized individual responsibility and market-driven solutions. This cultural framework shapes public attitudes, making the idea of a government-run healthcare system a hard sell for many Americans. Polls consistently show a nation divided, with support for single-payer healthcare varying widely based on political affiliation, age, and socioeconomic status.

At the political level, the single-payer debate has become a litmus test for ideological purity within the Democratic Party, while remaining a rallying point for opposition among Republicans. Progressive Democrats advocate for Medicare for All as a cornerstone of their platform, framing it as a moral and economic necessity. Moderates, however, caution against alienating voters who may view single-payer healthcare as too radical. Republicans, meanwhile, use the specter of single-payer healthcare to galvanize their base, warning of increased taxes and government control. This polarization ensures that single-payer healthcare remains a contentious and divisive issue, with little room for bipartisan compromise.

The debate also underscores the challenges of aligning a diverse and fragmented nation behind a unified vision of healthcare. In states like California and Vermont, where progressive ideals hold sway, single-payer proposals have gained traction but faced insurmountable obstacles in implementation. Funding mechanisms, legal challenges, and the logistical complexities of transitioning to a new system have repeatedly derailed state-level efforts, highlighting the practical difficulties of enacting single-payer healthcare even in supportive environments.

Moreover, the single-payer debate is complicated by the question of who benefits and who bears the cost. While universal coverage promises to address disparities in access to care, the transition to a single-payer system would likely involve significant disruption for those currently covered under employer-sponsored insurance. These individuals, who make up the majority of insured Americans, may be reluctant to trade their existing plans for the uncertainty of a new system. The financial burden of single-payer healthcare, which would require substantial tax increases, further complicates the calculus, particularly for middle- and upper-income households that may perceive themselves as net contributors rather than beneficiaries.

Despite these challenges, the single-payer debate continues to gain momentum, driven by growing dissatisfaction with the current system. Rising healthcare costs, mounting medical debt, and persistent disparities in access and outcomes fuel the argument that incremental reforms are no longer sufficient. For many Americans, the status quo is untenable, and single-payer healthcare represents a bold alternative that promises to address systemic failures. However, the path to such a transformation is fraught with obstacles, requiring not only a political realignment but also a cultural shift in how Americans perceive healthcare and its role in society.

Ultimately, the single-payer debate is a microcosm of the broader tensions that define American politics and society. It is a battle between competing visions of justice, freedom, and the role of government—a debate that transcends healthcare to touch on the very essence of what it means to be American. Whether single-payer healthcare can overcome the forces arrayed against it remains an open question, but the debate itself is a testament to the nation's struggle to reconcile its ideals with its realities. In this sense, the single-payer debate is not just about healthcare; it is about the future of America's social contract and the values that will define it in the years to come.

WHO BENEFITS FROM RHETORIC OVER REFORM?

The persistence of healthcare reform debates in the United States—marked by impassioned rhetoric but little substantive change—raises an uncomfortable question: who benefits from maintaining the illusion of progress without the reality of reform? At first glance, the absence of sweeping systemic change may seem like a failure of leadership or a consequence of political gridlock, but a closer examination reveals a more calculated dynamic. The healthcare system, as it currently operates, is not merely a fragmented and inefficient network; it is a multi-trillion-dollar ecosystem in which entrenched stakeholders have significant vested interests in preserving the status quo. These actors thrive in a climate of perpetual debate, using the guise of reform to protect their power, profits, and influence.

Foremost among these stakeholders are the private insurance companies, pharmaceutical giants, and hospital conglomerates that dominate the healthcare landscape. For these entities, the rhetoric of reform is a strategic tool, not a threat. By engaging in discussions of change—often in the form of nominal policy adjustments or pilot programs—they maintain the appearance of responsiveness while ensuring that fundamental disruptions to their business models are avoided. For example, proposals to expand access to insurance through public-private partnerships or incremental Medicare expansions often serve as compromises that leave the core profit-generating mechanisms of the private sector intact. The resulting inertia benefits these corporations by preventing the kind of radical overhaul—such as single-payer healthcare—that could undermine their economic dominance.

Pharmaceutical companies are another key beneficiary of the status quo, using the healthcare debate to deflect attention from practices that drive up drug prices while positioning themselves as innovators crucial to the system's success. While public outrage over exorbitant drug costs periodically flares, the industry counters with aggressive lobbying efforts, public relations campaigns, and minor concessions designed to appease critics without threatening their profit margins. Measures such as limited price caps on specific drugs or voluntary discount programs for certain patient groups create the illusion of progress while leaving the broader pricing structure untouched. The result is a system in which reform rhetoric pacifies public demands without addressing the underlying market forces that sustain exorbitant costs.

Politicians, too, derive significant benefits from the cyclical nature of healthcare debates. For those in office, healthcare reform serves as a reliable platform for galvanizing support, energizing their base, and framing themselves as champions of the people. However, the political incentives for actual reform are far weaker than those for perpetuating the debate. Sweeping changes to the system carry significant political risks: alienating powerful donors, provoking backlash from affected constituents, and inviting criticism from ideological opponents. By contrast, endorsing incremental reforms or vague aspirational goals allows politicians to maintain public support without incurring these costs. Campaign promises of universal healthcare or affordable prescription drugs, even when left unfulfilled, often suffice to sustain voter loyalty, creating a cycle in which rhetoric becomes a substitute for action.

Moreover, the healthcare debate serves as a political weapon, particularly in an era of heightened polarization. For conservatives, the specter of "socialized medicine" is a rallying cry against what they frame as government overreach, while progressives leverage the promise of Medicare for All to mobilize grassroots support and pressure moderates within their own party. This polarization ensures that the debate remains ideologically charged, making bipartisan solutions nearly impossible. In this environment, the rhetoric of reform functions less as a means of achieving consensus and more as a tool for consolidating political power.

In addition to corporate and political actors, an extensive ecosystem of intermediaries, consultants, and advocacy organizations profits from the endless cycle of healthcare debate. These groups—ranging from think tanks to lobbying firms—occupy a lucrative niche, shaping the conversation and influencing policy while benefiting from the lack of resolution. For example, consultants hired to navigate the complexities of the system or to advocate for specific reforms are often financially dependent on the very inefficiencies and ambiguities they claim to address. Similarly, advocacy organizations, while ostensibly working toward systemic change, often rely on the continuation of the debate to sustain their funding and relevance.

The media also plays a crucial role in perpetuating the cycle of rhetoric over reform. Complex discussions of healthcare policy are often reduced to soundbites, sensational headlines, or partisan talking points, making it easier to stoke outrage than to foster understanding. Coverage that frames healthcare reform as a zero-sum battle between opposing ideologies generates clicks, ratings, and advertising revenue, even as it deepens divisions and reinforces the status quo. In this environment, public discourse around healthcare becomes reactive rather than constructive, dominated by fear, misinformation, and emotional appeals rather than substantive analysis.

Meanwhile, ordinary Americans—those who ostensibly stand to benefit most from meaningful reform—are left navigating a system that prioritizes profits over patients. The rhetorical focus on access, affordability, and quality often masks the lived realities of a system in which millions remain uninsured, underinsured, or burdened by medical debt. These individuals become pawns in the broader debate, their struggles invoked as justifications for reform but rarely addressed in ways that lead to tangible improvements. Instead, the burden of navigating the fragmented system falls squarely on their shoulders, perpetuating cycles of inequality and suffering while powerful stakeholders profit from the inertia.

The dynamic of rhetoric over reform is not an accidental byproduct of dysfunction but a reflection of deliberate strategies employed by those who benefit from the status quo. By engaging in debates that promise progress but deliver little, these actors effectively neutralize threats to their interests while maintaining a veneer of responsiveness. The result is a system in which the appearance of reform becomes a substitute for actual change, ensuring that the forces of inertia prevail even as public dissatisfaction grows. For those at the helm of this system, the business of healthcare reform is not about solving problems but about managing perceptions—an endeavor that continues to pay dividends at the expense of those it purports to serve.

BREAKING THE CYCLE

Breaking the cycle of unfulfilled healthcare reform requires a paradigm shift that confronts the entrenched structures and systemic incentives perpetuating the status quo. For decades, reform has been framed as a question of incremental adjustments versus sweeping overhauls, a dichotomy that fails to address the deeper cultural, political, and economic forces at play. To escape this cycle, the first step is to redefine the parameters of the healthcare debate, shifting focus from short-term fixes to transformative solutions rooted in equity, accountability, and long-term sustainability.

Central to breaking this cycle is dismantling the financial and political stranglehold that corporate stakeholders maintain over the system. As long as insurance companies, pharmaceutical manufacturers, and hospital conglomerates dominate the healthcare agenda, the likelihood of meaningful reform remains slim. These entities exert influence not only through lobbying and campaign financing but also by shaping public narratives around what is feasible or desirable. Challenging their power requires implementing robust checks, such as strict campaign finance reforms, transparency in pricing, and caps on lobbying expenditures. By reducing the outsized influence of these stakeholders, policymakers can begin to reclaim the healthcare debate as one driven by public interest rather than profit.

Equally important is addressing the political dysfunction that sustains the cycle of rhetoric. The polarization of healthcare debates has created a zero-sum game in which compromise is framed as defeat, and ideological purity outweighs practical solutions. Breaking this dynamic requires fostering a culture of bipartisan collaboration, incentivizing coalition-building over party loyalty. This could involve structural changes, such as mandating cross-party committees to oversee healthcare reform or introducing ranked-choice voting systems that reward candidates who build consensus. Additionally, political leaders must be held accountable for turning campaign promises into actionable policies, a process that may involve more rigorous oversight mechanisms or citizen-led initiatives to track legislative progress.

A key obstacle to transformative reform is public disengagement, fueled by the complexity of the healthcare system and the cynicism bred by decades of unfulfilled promises. Breaking the cycle requires a concerted effort to educate and empower the public, making the healthcare system more accessible and understandable. This involves demystifying the intricacies of insurance plans, medical billing, and policy proposals, equipping citizens with the knowledge needed to advocate for change. Grassroots movements, community-based education programs, and digital platforms can play a vital role in mobilizing public support and ensuring that the voices of patients, caregivers, and underserved populations are at the forefront of the debate.

Moreover, breaking the cycle demands confronting the cultural narratives that have historically undermined reform efforts, particularly the deeply ingrained fear of government overreach. The demonization of state intervention in healthcare, perpetuated through decades of political rhetoric, has stymied progress by framing universal coverage as synonymous with inefficiency or loss of individual freedom. To counteract this, proponents of reform must reframe the narrative, highlighting the moral and economic imperative of a system that prioritizes collective well-being. Case studies from other nations, showcasing the successes and challenges of universal systems, can help illustrate the feasibility of reform while debunking misconceptions about its implications.

One of the most promising avenues for breaking the cycle lies in technological innovation, which has the potential to disrupt existing structures and introduce efficiencies previously thought unattainable. However, technology alone cannot address the inequities and systemic flaws embedded in the healthcare system. The integration of digital health tools, artificial intelligence, and telemedicine must be guided by ethical frameworks that prioritize accessibility, patient outcomes, and data privacy over profit motives. Public investment in technology infrastructure, coupled with policies that regulate its use, can ensure that innovation serves as a catalyst for reform rather than another tool for exploitation.

Finally, breaking the cycle requires a long-term vision that transcends electoral cycles and immediate political gains. Reform must be viewed not as a one-time achievement but as an ongoing process that evolves alongside societal needs and advancements in medical science. This entails establishing independent oversight bodies to monitor progress, adapt policies, and ensure that the system remains responsive to emerging challenges. By embedding adaptability into the framework of reform, policymakers can create a system capable of continuous improvement rather than periodic crisis management.

The challenge of breaking the healthcare reform cycle is formidable, given the entrenched interests and deep-seated narratives that sustain it. Yet, history has shown that transformative change is possible when public demand aligns with visionary leadership and systemic accountability. The task at hand is not merely to fix a broken system but to reimagine it, creating a healthcare model that reflects the values of justice, compassion, and shared responsibility. To do so requires not just addressing the symptoms of dysfunction but confronting its root causes, paving the way for a system that works for all, not just for those who profit from its failures.

Part 4: The Future of Healthcare in America

Chapter 10: The Role of Technology – A Cure or a Band-Aid?

Technology in healthcare exists within a space of profound contradiction. On one hand, it is heralded as the great equalizer, a means to expand access, enhance efficiency, and push the boundaries of medical science. On the other, it often acts as a mirror for the inequities already embedded in the healthcare system, amplifying existing disparities while introducing new ones. The narrative surrounding innovation tends to highlight its triumphs—the promise of artificial intelligence to diagnose diseases earlier than ever before, the convenience of telemedicine connecting patients in remote areas with specialists, and the vast potential of data analytics to predict and prevent public health crises. These are not small achievements; they represent a reimagining of what modern medicine can achieve when paired with technological ingenuity. Yet beneath these breakthroughs lies a troubling reality: technology in the U.S. healthcare system is shaped and constrained by the same market forces and structural inequalities that govern the rest of the industry.

The paradox of technology is most visible in how it creates winners and losers, often reinforcing the divide between those who can access cutting-edge advancements and those who are left behind. Telemedicine, for instance, surged during the COVID-19 pandemic as a lifeline for patients unable to visit healthcare facilities. For individuals with stable internet connections, private insurance, and the ability to navigate digital platforms, telemedicine was a revelation, offering unprecedented convenience and efficiency. But for others—those in rural areas with limited broadband access, older adults unfamiliar with the technology, and low-income families without the necessary devices—it remained out of reach. Similarly, artificial intelligence has demonstrated remarkable potential in improving diagnostics and treatment, but it often relies on data sets that fail to account for the diversity of the U.S. population, leading to biased outcomes that disproportionately harm marginalized communities.

Even the promise of data-driven care, with its ability to harness vast troves of information to personalize treatment and optimize outcomes, is complicated by issues of privacy, accessibility, and corporate control. Healthcare technology companies increasingly act as custodians of patient data, raising questions about who truly benefits from these innovations. Are they designed to serve the public good, or do they prioritize profitability and market dominance? These questions underscore the central tension of a profit-driven healthcare system: the potential of technology to revolutionize care is inevitably filtered through the lens of financial viability and return on investment.

This paradox is not a reflection of technological failure but of systemic design. In a system where healthcare is treated as a commodity rather than a universal right, the tools of innovation often exacerbate existing divides rather than bridging them. Technology, for all its promise, cannot operate in a vacuum. It is shaped by the policies, structures, and ideologies that govern its deployment, and in the U.S., this means its potential is often constrained by the imperatives of the market. Far from being an inherent flaw of the technology itself, this reality is a symptom of a deeper systemic issue: a healthcare system that prioritizes profitability over equity, innovation over inclusion. As a result, technology becomes a double-edged sword, capable of both profound progress and deepening inequity, a cure for some and a mere band-aid for others.

THE PROMISES OF TECHNOLOGY IN HEALTHCARE

The promises of technology in healthcare are vast and undeniably transformative, offering solutions to some of the most persistent challenges in modern medicine. Artificial intelligence holds the potential to reshape diagnostics, identifying diseases with a precision and speed that even the most skilled physicians struggle to match. Machine learning algorithms, trained on millions of cases, can detect subtle patterns in medical imaging or genetic data, catching cancers, heart conditions, or rare diseases long before symptoms become critical. For those fortunate enough to access these tools, AI promises not only earlier interventions but more personalized treatment plans tailored to the unique biology of each patient. The efficiencies introduced by AI extend beyond clinical care, streamlining administrative processes, reducing waste, and cutting through the bureaucratic bottlenecks that plague the healthcare system.

Telemedicine, which saw a dramatic expansion during the COVID-19 pandemic, offers another compelling vision of the future. By enabling patients to consult with doctors remotely, it eliminates the barriers of geography, saving time and reducing the burden on overtaxed healthcare facilities. For rural communities, where specialist care is often hours away, telemedicine has the potential to deliver life-saving consultations and continuous care to populations that have long been neglected. It transforms the notion of accessibility, bringing care into the homes of patients who might otherwise forego treatment due to logistical challenges or physical limitations.

Data-driven care is another frontier of immense promise. The ability to analyze vast quantities of patient data has already begun to redefine public health, identifying trends, predicting outbreaks, and informing policy decisions with unprecedented precision. On an individual level, predictive analytics can flag high-risk patients, allowing for targeted interventions before minor health issues become catastrophic. The integration of wearable technology—devices that monitor heart rates, blood pressure, glucose levels, or sleep patterns—further personalizes care, empowering patients to manage their health proactively while providing physicians with real-time insights. These advancements suggest a future where medicine is not only reactive but anticipatory, a shift that could reduce suffering and dramatically lower costs.

The most optimistic narratives around healthcare technology position it as the great equalizer, capable of extending high-quality care to all regardless of socioeconomic status, geography, or demographic profile. In theory, these innovations could break down traditional barriers, bringing precision medicine to underserved communities, reducing human error in diagnosis, and making care more efficient and effective across the board. The potential for these tools to save lives, improve quality of care, and drive down costs is undeniable. For policymakers and providers, they represent an alluring promise: a way to address inefficiencies in the system without the need for sweeping structural reforms. For patients, they symbolize hope—an assurance that healthcare is evolving in ways that could deliver better outcomes and more humane treatment.

Yet, as dazzling as these promises may appear, they cannot be divorced from the realities of their implementation. The potential for technology to revolutionize healthcare exists not in isolation but within a system where access, affordability, and equity remain unresolved issues. These tools may redefine what is possible in medicine, but the question remains: for whom will this progress truly matter? The promise of technology in healthcare, while extraordinary, is ultimately contingent on the structures within which it operates. Without addressing the underlying inequities of the system, even the most advanced innovations risk falling short of their transformative potential.

The Limitations of Technological Solutions

While the promises of healthcare technology are compelling, their limitations reveal the systemic challenges and inequities that continue to shape their implementation. Technology, for all its advancements, does not exist in a vacuum; it operates within a healthcare framework deeply influenced by market forces, profit motives, and uneven access. As a result, its benefits are often unevenly distributed, with the very innovations designed to enhance care creating new barriers for those already marginalized.

Artificial intelligence, hailed for its diagnostic precision, is not immune to the biases of the data it relies upon. AI systems are only as effective as the datasets they are trained on, and many of these datasets fail to adequately represent diverse populations. This can lead to diagnostic errors or outright exclusion for racial and ethnic minorities, women, or those with uncommon conditions. An algorithm trained primarily on data from affluent, insured patients may perform poorly when applied to populations with different genetic backgrounds or environmental exposures. In such cases, rather than addressing disparities, AI risks entrenching them, perpetuating systemic inequalities under the guise of innovation.

Telemedicine, similarly, illustrates the gap between promise and reality. While it has brought convenience to many, its reliance on stable internet connections, access to digital devices, and technological literacy creates significant barriers for vulnerable populations. Rural communities, ironically among those who could benefit most from remote care, often lack the broadband infrastructure necessary to support telemedicine platforms. Older adults, who frequently suffer from chronic conditions requiring consistent medical oversight, may struggle to navigate unfamiliar technologies or lack access to smartphones or computers. Telemedicine, far from bridging the gap in access, can inadvertently widen it, leaving those in greatest need even further behind.

Data-driven care, for all its analytical potential, also raises pressing ethical and logistical concerns. The aggregation and analysis of patient data are often controlled by private companies whose primary obligation is to shareholders, not patients. Questions about privacy, consent, and data security become paramount in a system where sensitive health information is treated as a commodity. Moreover, the insights generated by these data analytics are frequently leveraged to optimize profits rather than improve outcomes for all. For example, insurers may use predictive algorithms to identify high-cost patients, not to enhance their care, but to deny coverage or increase premiums.

The integration of wearable technology highlights another dimension of these limitations: the burden of responsibility placed on patients themselves. While these devices empower individuals to monitor their own health, they also create an implicit expectation that patients will take full accountability for managing conditions, often without the support or resources necessary to do so effectively. For low-income patients, the cost of wearable devices or subscription-based health apps can be prohibitive, making these tools a luxury rather than a universally accessible solution.

Perhaps the most profound limitation of technological solutions lies in their inability to address the root causes of inequity in the healthcare system. Technology can optimize processes, enhance diagnostics, and expand the reach of care, but it cannot correct for systemic underfunding of public health initiatives, the lack of universal coverage, or the profit-driven motives that prioritize innovation for the wealthy over basic care for the underserved. Instead of serving as a great equalizer, technology often becomes a reflection of the inequalities already present in the system, amplifying advantages for those who can afford them while offering little relief to those who cannot.

These limitations underscore a sobering truth: technology, for all its transformative potential, is not a panacea. Its effectiveness is inherently constrained by the environment in which it is deployed. In the U.S. healthcare system, where access to care is deeply stratified and market imperatives drive decision-making, technology frequently serves as a band-aid rather than a cure—a tool to enhance care for some while leaving systemic inequities untouched or exacerbated. To realize its full potential, technology must be paired with structural reforms that address the underlying disparities that continue to define the landscape of American healthcare.

THE DIVIDE BETWEEN WINNERS AND LOSERS

The integration of technology into the U.S. healthcare system has created a sharp divide between winners and losers, amplifying the disparities inherent in a system driven by profit and privilege. While the beneficiaries of these advancements—often those with wealth, stable insurance, and access to elite healthcare providers—celebrate a new era of personalized, efficient care, others are left grappling with the widening chasm of inequity. Technology, rather than leveling the playing field, frequently reinforces the barriers that separate those who can access its promises from those who cannot.

The winners of this technological revolution are clear. Affluent patients gain access to state-of-the-art diagnostic tools, precision medicine tailored to their genetic profiles, and concierge telemedicine services that bring physicians to their devices at a moment's notice. These individuals navigate a healthcare system augmented by AI-driven platforms that reduce wait times, streamline administrative processes, and connect them to cutting-edge treatments. For this segment of the population, technology has transformed healthcare into a seamless, responsive experience—a demonstration of the system's capacity to innovate and improve outcomes when financial limitations are removed.

Providers and corporations are also among the winners. Hospitals and private practices that can afford to adopt advanced technologies position themselves as leaders in the field, attracting patients and investors alike. Pharmaceutical companies use data analytics to identify lucrative markets for new drugs, while insurers harness predictive algorithms to optimize risk management. These players leverage technology not only to improve efficiency but also to maximize profitability, often at the expense of equitable access.

For the losers, however, the story is starkly different. Low-income patients, rural residents, and marginalized communities are often excluded from these technological advancements due to systemic barriers. Telemedicine, for instance, holds little value for those without reliable internet access or digital devices. Rural hospitals, which serve as lifelines for underserved communities, frequently lack the resources to invest in cutting-edge technologies, leaving their patients reliant on outdated systems. The promise of AI-driven diagnostics is meaningless to those without insurance or the ability to afford the expensive tests these tools often recommend.

This divide is particularly visible in the growing reliance on wearable technology and data-driven health interventions. Affluent individuals can afford smartwatches and continuous monitoring devices that provide early warnings for potential health issues, while lower-income patients often lack access to even basic preventive care. The benefits of personalized medicine, enabled by genomic testing and advanced analytics, are similarly restricted to those who can pay for the privilege. These innovations, hailed as breakthroughs in modern medicine, remain out of reach for the very populations that could benefit most from early intervention and targeted treatment.

The divide extends beyond patients to healthcare workers themselves. Physicians and nurses in well-funded institutions are increasingly equipped with AI tools and streamlined workflows that reduce their burden and enhance their decision-making. In contrast, those working in underfunded or rural facilities face the dual challenge of outdated infrastructure and overwhelming patient loads. The lack of technological resources compounds their stress and exacerbates burnout, further straining the fragile safety net these workers are meant to uphold.

The broader implications of this divide are profound. By concentrating the benefits of technological advancements among the privileged, the U.S. healthcare system perpetuates a two-tiered model of care—one defined by innovation and abundance, the other by scarcity and neglect. The very tools designed to improve efficiency and outcomes risk becoming symbols of exclusion, serving as reminders of the structural inequities that define the system. As technology accelerates the pace of medical progress, it also accelerates the pace at which disparities deepen, challenging the narrative that innovation alone can solve the healthcare system's most pressing problems. Without deliberate efforts to democratize access and address systemic barriers, the gap between healthcare's winners and losers will continue to grow, reinforcing a hierarchy of care that leaves the most vulnerable further behind.

Ethical and Policy Implications

The ethical and policy implications of a profit-driven, technology-infused healthcare system reveal the deep tensions between innovation, equity, and accountability. At the heart of these tensions lies a question that has long haunted the U.S. healthcare system: Should access to life-saving or life-improving technology be a privilege based on market dynamics, or a right ensured through deliberate policy interventions? This dilemma shapes every aspect of how technology is developed, deployed, and experienced, often to the detriment of those who are least equipped to navigate its complexities.

Ethically, the commercialization of healthcare technologies raises profound concerns about justice and fairness. When cutting-edge innovations—whether AI-driven diagnostics, personalized medicine, or telehealth platforms—are disproportionately accessible to wealthier, insured populations, the system implicitly prioritizes profits over patient welfare. This creates a moral paradox: technologies developed to save lives and improve health are monetized in ways that restrict their benefits to those who can pay. The ethical principles of beneficence and justice are subordinated to market imperatives, leaving millions without access to tools that could dramatically improve their health outcomes.

This inequity is exacerbated by the privatization of health data. Patients often have little say over how their medical information is collected, stored, and used by corporations that profit from it. Data-driven insights, which could be harnessed to address systemic disparities, are instead channeled into optimizing revenue streams for insurers, pharmaceutical companies, and healthcare providers. The commodification of health data also raises critical concerns about privacy and consent. When algorithms are built on proprietary data sets controlled by private entities, the public has limited visibility into how decisions about their care are made, further eroding trust in the system.

On a policy level, these ethical dilemmas are compounded by a regulatory environment that has struggled to keep pace with technological innovation. The rapid adoption of AI in healthcare, for example, has outstripped the development of clear guidelines for accountability and oversight. When algorithms make diagnostic errors or perpetuate biases, who is held responsible? Is it the developer, the provider, or the institution that adopted the technology? These unanswered questions highlight the need for robust policy frameworks that balance the drive for innovation with safeguards to protect patients from harm and ensure equitable access.

The lack of universal healthcare in the U.S. adds another layer of complexity to the policy landscape. Unlike nations with single-payer systems, where new technologies are evaluated for their cost-effectiveness and societal benefit before broad implementation, the U.S. leaves much of this decision-making to market forces. This results in a patchwork of access, where technological adoption is determined by profitability rather than public health priorities. Policy efforts to bridge this gap—such as expanding Medicare coverage for telehealth services—often fall short of addressing the structural inequalities that underpin the system.

Moreover, the reliance on for-profit entities to drive technological innovation creates an inherent conflict of interest. Pharmaceutical companies, for instance, invest heavily in developing new treatments, but their pricing strategies often put these therapies out of reach for many patients. Similarly, hospitals and health systems that invest in expensive AI tools or robotic surgical devices are incentivized to focus on high-margin procedures that cater to affluent patients, rather than deploying these technologies in underserved areas where they might have the greatest public health impact.

These ethical and policy implications demand a reevaluation of the role technology plays in healthcare. Policymakers must grapple with how to democratize access to technological advancements while preserving the incentives that drive innovation. This will require bold interventions, such as subsidies for rural hospitals adopting telemedicine, stricter regulations on the use of patient data, and incentives for developers to prioritize equity in their algorithms and technologies. Ethical frameworks must evolve to hold corporations accountable for the societal impacts of their innovations, ensuring that the pursuit of profit does not come at the expense of patient welfare or the public good.

The profit-driven integration of technology into healthcare reflects the broader values of the U.S. system—innovation and competition, yes, but also exclusion and inequity. The ethical and policy challenges it presents are not technological in nature but systemic, rooted in a model that prioritizes market efficiency over universal access. Addressing these challenges will require a shift not only in how technology is developed and deployed but in how the healthcare system as a whole conceptualizes its obligations to those it serves. Without this shift, the ethical promises of technology will remain as elusive as the policy solutions needed to fulfill them, leaving the U.S. healthcare system trapped in a cycle of innovation without equity.

Technology as a Complement, Not a Cure

Despite its transformative potential, technology in healthcare must be understood as a complement to human expertise, institutional reform, and social investment rather than a standalone cure for systemic dysfunction. The allure of technological solutions often lies in their promise to bypass entrenched challenges with innovation, offering efficiency, precision, and scalability. However, this promise, while compelling, risks obscuring the fundamental structural issues that technology alone cannot resolve. It is neither a panacea for inequity nor a substitute for comprehensive policy changes; rather, it functions best when integrated into a broader framework of care designed to balance innovation with accessibility.

Healthcare, at its core, is a profoundly human endeavor, requiring empathy, judgment, and trust—qualities that no algorithm, however sophisticated, can replicate. AI may enhance diagnostic accuracy, and telemedicine may bridge geographic gaps, but neither can address the deeply personal and social aspects of care that rely on interpersonal connection. A patient suffering from chronic illness does not only need an accurate diagnosis; they need a provider who listens, understands their unique circumstances, and collaborates on a feasible treatment plan. When technology is deployed without considering these relational dimensions, it risks reducing patients to data points and care to transactions.

Moreover, technology's potential is inherently limited by the context in which it operates. In a fragmented and profit-driven healthcare system, even the most advanced innovations can perpetuate or exacerbate disparities. Telemedicine, for example, cannot resolve the lack of broadband access in rural areas or the language barriers faced by immigrant communities. AI-driven tools may identify risk factors with incredible precision, but they cannot overcome systemic barriers such as unaffordable medications or inadequate insurance coverage. These tools can complement care by optimizing certain processes, but they cannot substitute for the investments needed to address the root causes of healthcare inequity.

Policymakers and healthcare leaders must resist the temptation to overestimate technology's role in solving these deeper issues. For every success story of AI diagnosing rare diseases or robotic surgery minimizing patient recovery times, there are countless examples where technology failed to deliver meaningful improvement due to implementation challenges, cost barriers, or institutional resistance. Technology, no matter how advanced, requires infrastructure, training, and adaptation to local contexts to succeed. When these factors are neglected, the most well-intentioned innovations can falter, leaving underserved populations further behind.

The profit motives driving technological development also underscore the necessity of treating these tools as complements rather than cures. Many innovations are designed with profitability, not universality, in mind. High-cost treatments, wearable health devices, and personalized medicine often target affluent markets, sidelining broader public health needs. Even when new technologies have the potential to benefit all, their deployment is often dictated by financial incentives rather than societal priorities. Without deliberate efforts to align technological advancements with public health goals, their impact will remain limited to the privileged few.

To harness the true potential of technology in healthcare, it must be integrated into a system that prioritizes equitable access and human-centered care. This requires policies that incentivize not only the development of advanced tools but also their deployment in underserved areas. It calls for investments in the social determinants of health—education, housing, nutrition—that no algorithm can address but that profoundly influence health outcomes. It demands a rethinking of healthcare delivery models to ensure that technology augments rather than replaces the human relationships that define effective care.

When viewed as a complement rather than a cure, technology can be a powerful force for good. It can streamline administrative burdens, freeing providers to focus on patient care. It can expand access to specialized expertise in remote areas, bringing high-quality care to those who need it most. It can generate insights from vast amounts of data, enabling public health interventions that save lives on a large scale. But these benefits will only be realized if technology is deployed thoughtfully, within a system that values equity as much as efficiency.

In the end, the promise of healthcare technology lies not in its ability to revolutionize the system on its own but in its capacity to enhance the work of dedicated providers, strengthen the reach of public health initiatives, and address specific gaps in access and care. By recognizing its limitations and embracing its role as part of a broader, more holistic approach, technology can help build a healthcare system that is not only innovative but also just, sustainable, and humane.

Chapter 11: Privatization vs. Universal Care – What's Next?

The debate between privatization and universal care reflects a profound ideological schism about the nature of healthcare itself: Is it a commodity to be bought and sold, or a fundamental right to be guaranteed? Privatization champions the efficiencies of market-driven systems, claiming they spur innovation, reduce costs through competition, and offer consumers greater choice. Proponents of universal care counter these claims by framing healthcare as a public good, emphasizing the moral imperative of equitable access and the long-term benefits of healthier populations.

At its core, privatization relies on the premise that markets function best when minimally constrained, with price signals guiding the efficient allocation of resources. Advocates argue that private insurers, hospitals, and pharmaceutical companies thrive under competition, incentivized to innovate and cater to consumer needs. Yet, in the U.S., the heavy reliance on private actors has produced outcomes that challenge this optimistic vision: the highest healthcare costs among developed nations, inconsistent quality, and glaring disparities in access. Critics point to these failures as evidence of systemic dysfunction, arguing that the profit motive in healthcare can lead to perverse incentives, where financial interests outweigh patient well-being.

Universal care, in contrast, posits that the collective pooling of resources enables societies to prioritize health equity and public welfare. By eliminating profit motives from basic healthcare delivery, universal systems aim to reduce administrative inefficiencies, cap costs, and ensure that no one is excluded due to inability to pay. Yet, detractors warn of bureaucratic inefficiency, reduced innovation, and the potential for rationing care. These criticisms, while not unfounded, often rest on selective interpretations of universal systems, ignoring their capacity to deliver superior outcomes in terms of life expectancy, infant mortality, and patient satisfaction compared to privatized models.

The U.S. healthcare debate is uniquely charged, shaped by cultural narratives of individualism, freedom, and mistrust of government intervention. This ideological backdrop complicates reform efforts, making healthcare policy as much about identity as about pragmatism. Attempts to expand public programs or regulate private markets are frequently framed as existential threats to personal liberty, while the human cost of a fragmented and expensive system often fades into abstraction. In this polarized context, both privatization and universal care represent not only different policy options but competing visions of what society owes its citizens.

Increased Privatization: Efficiency or Exclusion?

The push for increased privatization in healthcare often comes with promises of greater efficiency, innovation, and responsiveness to consumer demands. Proponents argue that private markets thrive on competition, driving down costs while improving the quality of services. The vision is one of a sleek, customer-centered healthcare system where patients can shop for coverage or services like any other product, empowered by transparency in pricing and quality metrics. Yet this optimistic portrayal often obscures the underlying realities of what privatization entails and whom it ultimately serves.

Efficiency in privatized systems, while plausible in theory, frequently translates into cost-cutting measures that prioritize profit over patient outcomes. Administrative overhead, marketing expenses, and shareholder dividends absorb significant portions of healthcare spending, diverting resources away from direct patient care. Cost-saving strategies, such as network restrictions or preauthorization requirements, may limit access to necessary treatments, leaving patients entangled in bureaucratic processes that delay or deny care. Critics contend that such practices erode trust in the system, fostering resentment and skepticism toward insurers and providers alike.

Moreover, privatization often intensifies healthcare inequalities. Those with financial means can access premium services, while marginalized populations are left to navigate fragmented and underfunded options. For example, high-deductible health plans, hailed as cost-containment tools, shift financial risk onto patients, disproportionately affecting those with chronic illnesses or lower incomes. In rural and underserved areas, the retreat of private entities, deemed unprofitable, creates healthcare deserts where even basic services are scarce.

Privatization's promise of choice is thus revealed as an illusion for many, constrained by systemic barriers that favor wealthier individuals and urban centers.

The exclusionary tendencies of privatized systems also extend to the workforce. As private entities seek to maximize efficiency, they often impose rigid cost controls on clinicians, increasing workloads while reducing autonomy. Burnout among healthcare workers, already a critical issue, is exacerbated by these pressures, leading to higher turnover and diminished quality of care. Patients and providers alike find themselves ensnared in a system optimized for profitability rather than health outcomes, with long-term societal costs that far outweigh short-term savings.

Finally, the ethical dimension of privatization cannot be ignored. By framing healthcare as a commodity rather than a right, privatization implicitly endorses a system where the ability to pay determines access to life-saving services. For many, this approach is fundamentally at odds with the principles of justice and human dignity. The question, then, is whether efficiency gained through privatization—assuming it is achieved—justifies the exclusion it perpetuates, or whether a society can afford to accept a system where market forces dictate the boundaries of care.

The Hybrid Model: Balancing Market and Public Goals

The hybrid model, blending elements of privatization with public healthcare provisions, has emerged as a pragmatic approach in countries seeking to balance the efficiency of markets with the equity of state-driven systems. Proponents of this model argue that it offers the best of both worlds: the innovation and responsiveness of private enterprise combined with the accessibility and protections afforded by public oversight. However, achieving such a balance is a delicate and often fraught endeavor, requiring continuous calibration to align market incentives with broader societal goals.

At its core, the hybrid model acknowledges the limitations of both extremes. Purely privatized systems risk excluding vulnerable populations, while wholly public systems often struggle with inefficiencies and resource constraints. By integrating these approaches, hybrid systems aim to harness the strengths of each. For instance, private insurers may be incentivized to compete on cost and quality within a regulatory framework that ensures universal coverage. Public programs, like Medicare or Medicaid, can serve as safety nets, while private options cater to those seeking supplementary or expedited care. This dual structure seeks to provide comprehensive access without stifling the dynamism of private innovation.

Yet, the hybrid approach is not without its challenges. One of its central tensions lies in reconciling the profit motives of private entities with the egalitarian objectives of public health policy. When private providers are tasked with delivering publicly funded services, conflicts of interest frequently arise. For example, profit-driven entities may prioritize low-cost, high-margin treatments over less lucrative but clinically necessary interventions. These dynamics can lead to fragmented care, with patients navigating a labyrinth of private and public options, each with distinct rules, pricing structures, and access criteria.

The hybrid model also faces structural inefficiencies that stem from its inherent complexity. Administrative costs tend to soar in systems where multiple payers coexist, each requiring distinct billing procedures, reimbursement models, and compliance standards. Patients, too, often bear the burden of this complexity, contending with opaque pricing, network limitations, and inconsistent coverage. Despite its promise of balance, the hybrid model risks reproducing some of the very inefficiencies it seeks to mitigate, challenging its capacity to deliver seamless, equitable care.

Furthermore, the hybrid model's success depends heavily on effective regulation and governance. Governments must establish clear frameworks to ensure that private actors align their practices with public health objectives. This entails setting reimbursement rates, enforcing quality standards, and preventing exploitative practices such as price gouging or service rationing. However, regulatory capture—the phenomenon where private entities exert undue influence over policymakers—poses a significant threat. When regulations are shaped to favor industry interests rather than public welfare, the hybrid model can devolve into a façade of balance, masking deep inequities and systemic flaws.

Despite these challenges, the hybrid model remains a compelling pathway for countries like the United States, where political and cultural resistance to both full privatization and universal care is deeply entrenched. Its potential lies in fostering incremental reform, leveraging market forces to drive innovation while safeguarding the principle that access to healthcare is a fundamental right. The success of this model ultimately hinges on the willingness of stakeholders—governments, corporations, providers, and the public—to commit to a shared vision of care that transcends profit margins and prioritizes human well-being.

STEPS TOWARD UNIVERSALITY: BRIDGING THE GAP

The journey toward universality in healthcare requires a multifaceted and pragmatic approach, one that seeks to bridge the ideological and systemic divides that have long characterized the U.S. healthcare system. Unlike radical upheavals, incremental steps toward universal coverage hold the greatest potential for garnering broad-based support while addressing the immediate needs of underserved populations. This pathway involves expanding access, addressing cost barriers, and establishing a cultural shift in the collective understanding of healthcare as a right rather than a privilege.

At the heart of this transition lies the need to fill existing gaps in coverage without dismantling the private sector infrastructure that millions of Americans currently rely upon. Programs like Medicaid and the Affordable Care Act (ACA) have already demonstrated the feasibility of expanding access through government intervention while maintaining a role for private insurers. Building on these frameworks, policymakers can consider initiatives such as automatic enrollment for uninsured individuals, subsidies to make private plans more affordable, or even a public option that allows citizens to choose between government-run insurance and private alternatives. These steps offer a pragmatic compromise, increasing coverage rates without alienating those who favor market-driven solutions.

Another critical component involves addressing the spiraling costs of care, which remain one of the most significant barriers to universality. Price transparency regulations, negotiated drug prices, and caps on out-of-pocket expenses are all measures that can help control costs while preserving choice and competition. The goal is to shift the focus of healthcare from profit maximization to patient-centered outcomes, creating a system where affordability is no longer synonymous with limited access. This reorientation would require robust federal oversight to ensure compliance and to prevent private entities from exploiting loopholes that perpetuate inequities.

Bridging the gap toward universality also demands a reimagining of preventive care as a cornerstone of the healthcare system. By prioritizing early interventions, wellness programs, and community health initiatives, the system can reduce the overall burden of chronic diseases that drive much of its inefficiency. Universal preventive care, supported by government funding, would not only lower costs but also foster a healthier population, reducing the dependency on reactive, high-cost treatments. Such measures align with both public health objectives and fiscal prudence, making them appealing across the political spectrum.

Cultural shifts are equally vital in paving the way for universality. In a society deeply rooted in individualism and market-based ideologies, the concept of healthcare as a shared societal responsibility often encounters resistance. Overcoming this obstacle requires concerted efforts to reframe the narrative around healthcare, emphasizing its role in ensuring economic productivity, social stability, and individual dignity. Public education campaigns, backed by data and personal stories, can help dispel myths about universal care while highlighting the human and economic costs of the status quo.

The path to universality hinges on political will and coalition-building. Achieving systemic change requires aligning diverse stakeholders, from policymakers and healthcare providers to patients and advocacy groups. The process will involve navigating entrenched interests, including powerful industry lobbies, and finding common ground between competing ideologies. While the obstacles are significant, history has shown that incremental progress can build momentum for larger reforms. Each step, however small, brings the system closer to the ideal of universality, where healthcare is accessible to all and reflective of a society's commitment to equity and compassion.

Obstacles to Systemic Overhaul in a Capitalist Society

The obstacles to systemic overhaul in the U.S. healthcare system are deeply rooted in the nation's economic framework and cultural ethos, which prioritize free-market capitalism over collective welfare. At the heart of these challenges lies a tension between profit-driven imperatives and the ethical obligation to ensure equitable access to healthcare. In a society where success is often measured by market competition and individual achievement, proposals for systemic change frequently encounter resistance from powerful stakeholders, ideological divisions, and deeply ingrained perceptions of government intervention.

One of the most formidable barriers to overhaul is the entrenched influence of private interests that dominate the healthcare industry. Insurance companies, pharmaceutical manufacturers, and hospital conglomerates wield immense political and economic power, leveraging extensive lobbying networks to preserve the status quo. These entities often frame reform efforts as threats to innovation, competition, and quality, despite evidence that their profit motives frequently inflate costs and limit access. Their financial contributions to political campaigns and advertising strategies enable them to shape public opinion and policymaking, creating a formidable wall against proposals perceived as undermining their economic interests.

Public skepticism toward government-run systems is another major obstacle. Decades of political rhetoric have framed universal healthcare as synonymous with inefficiency, higher taxes, and reduced choice. The specter of "socialized medicine" has been used to stoke fears of bureaucratic overreach, rationing, and declining quality, despite the success of universal systems in other developed nations. For many Americans, the belief that market competition inherently drives quality and innovation persists, even in the face of mounting evidence that the profit motive in healthcare often exacerbates inefficiencies and inequities.

The fragmented nature of the current system also poses logistical challenges to systemic overhaul. With a mix of private insurance, employer-sponsored plans, and government programs like Medicare and Medicaid, any effort to implement universal coverage would require reconciling these disparate elements. Transitioning to a single-payer or hybrid system would involve significant upheaval, including potential job losses in the insurance sector and complex adjustments to billing and payment infrastructures. The scale of such a transformation generates uncertainty and resistance, even among those who acknowledge the flaws of the current system.

Cultural attitudes toward individual responsibility and meritocracy further complicate reform efforts. In the U.S., healthcare is often seen as a commodity rather than a right, and the idea that individuals should earn access through employment or personal success is deeply ingrained. This perspective fosters resistance to collective solutions, as they are perceived to undermine personal accountability or redistribute resources in ways deemed unfair. Overcoming this cultural barrier requires shifting the narrative around healthcare, framing it not as a privilege but as a societal investment in human potential and dignity.

Finally, the political landscape is fraught with partisanship and gridlock, making consensus on healthcare reform extraordinarily difficult. Efforts to expand access or control costs are frequently weaponized as partisan issues, with opposing sides accusing each other of jeopardizing economic stability or human lives. This polarization not only stymies meaningful debate but also erodes public trust in the ability of government to enact effective change. The cyclical nature of elections further complicates long-term planning, as new administrations often prioritize undoing their predecessors' reforms rather than building on them.

The obstacles to systemic overhaul in a capitalist society are both structural and ideological, requiring more than just policy proposals to overcome. They demand a fundamental rethinking of the relationship between profit and care, a recalibration of cultural values, and a commitment to building coalitions that transcend partisan divides. While the path forward is fraught with challenges, acknowledging these barriers is the first step toward envisioning and enacting a healthcare system that serves all Americans more equitably and sustainably.

Comparative Insights: Lessons from Global Experiences

Comparative insights from global healthcare systems offer a valuable lens for understanding the possibilities and limitations of reforming the U.S. healthcare system. Examining models from countries that have implemented universal care, hybrid systems, or privatized approaches highlights both aspirational goals and cautionary tales. While no single model can be seamlessly transplanted into the U.S. due to its unique cultural, political, and economic context, these experiences provide a roadmap for addressing systemic inefficiencies, expanding access, and balancing market incentives with public welfare.

Universal care systems, such as those in Canada and the United Kingdom, underscore the potential benefits of prioritizing equity and access over profitability. In Canada, a single-payer model ensures that all citizens have access to necessary medical services, funded through taxation and delivered without financial barriers at the point of care. Similarly, the United Kingdom's National Health Service (NHS) operates as a government-run system that emphasizes preventive care and population health outcomes. These models achieve lower per capita healthcare spending and better health indicators compared to the U.S., demonstrating that universal coverage can coexist with cost efficiency. However, they also face challenges, including wait times for non-urgent procedures and resource constraints, which critics often cite as trade-offs for equity.

Hybrid systems, like those in Germany and the Netherlands, offer an alternative pathway that blends market mechanisms with universal coverage. In Germany, a multi-payer system combines statutory health insurance with private options, ensuring comprehensive care while allowing for individual choice. The Netherlands employs a regulated competition model, where private insurers compete within a framework of universal coverage mandates and government oversight. These systems demonstrate that markets can coexist with equity when carefully regulated, offering lessons for the U.S. on balancing competition with universal access. Yet, they also highlight the importance of strict regulation to prevent profit motives from undermining care quality or accessibility.

Privatized systems, such as Singapore's, show how targeted government intervention can coexist with market-driven healthcare. Singapore's model relies on mandatory savings accounts, known as Medisave, supplemented by government subsidies and catastrophic coverage. This approach emphasizes individual responsibility while providing a safety net for the most vulnerable, resulting in one of the most cost-effective healthcare systems globally. However, the cultural and economic differences between Singapore and the U.S. limit the direct applicability of this model. Singapore's smaller population and strong social cohesion enable policies that might face resistance in the more diverse and fragmented U.S. landscape.

The Nordic countries—Sweden, Denmark, and Norway—provide further insights into the role of government in healthcare. These nations prioritize public funding, transparency, and a commitment to reducing health disparities. Their systems integrate social determinants of health, such as education, housing, and nutrition, into broader policy frameworks, recognizing that healthcare outcomes are inseparable from societal conditions. This holistic approach offers a valuable lesson for the U.S., where addressing disparities often requires tackling upstream factors like poverty and systemic racism. However, the U.S.'s larger and more heterogeneous population presents challenges to implementing such comprehensive strategies on a national scale.

Lessons from global systems also illuminate potential pitfalls. Countries like Australia and New Zealand, which rely on hybrid models, have faced rising costs as private insurers expand their influence, creating disparities in access to advanced care. Even in systems that achieve universal coverage, balancing sustainability with rising healthcare demands remains a common challenge, particularly as populations age and chronic diseases increase.

The global landscape underscores that healthcare reform is not a one-size-fits-all endeavor. While universal and hybrid systems demonstrate that equity and efficiency are achievable, they also reveal that effective governance, cultural buy-in, and adaptable policies are essential for success. For the U.S., the comparative insights suggest that meaningful reform will require not only technical solutions but also a willingness to confront entrenched interests, rethink cultural narratives around healthcare, and address the systemic inequities that underpin the current system. In learning from the successes and challenges of other nations, the U.S. can chart a path toward a healthcare model that reflects both its values and its aspirations for a healthier, more equitable society.

FUTURE SCENARIOS: NAVIGATING THE CROSSROADS

The future of the U.S. healthcare system stands at a complex and contentious crossroads, shaped by competing visions of reform and the persistent challenges of balancing access, quality, and cost. The trajectory it takes will depend on decisions made at the intersection of politics, economics, and cultural values. Whether through deepened privatization, incremental hybrid adjustments, or a gradual shift toward universal care, each scenario carries profound implications for patients, providers, and policymakers alike.

Increased privatization represents one potential path, emphasizing market-driven solutions and the efficiencies they promise. Proponents argue that greater competition could lower costs, foster innovation, and streamline service delivery. This vision leans heavily on deregulation and the empowerment of private insurers, pharmaceutical companies, and healthcare providers to expand their reach. However, such a trajectory risks deepening existing inequities. Without sufficient safeguards, privatization could exacerbate disparities, leaving underserved communities and vulnerable populations further marginalized. Healthcare would increasingly be treated as a commodity, with access tied closely to income and employment stability.

A more likely path, given the deeply entrenched interests in the current system, involves incremental reforms within a hybrid framework. This scenario envisions pragmatic policy changes aimed at expanding coverage while retaining private sector involvement. Measures like enhancing the Affordable Care Act, offering a public option alongside private insurance, and capping out-of-pocket expenses could incrementally improve equity and affordability without fundamentally restructuring the system. While politically palatable, this approach runs the risk of entrenching inefficiencies, as piecemeal adjustments may fail to address systemic flaws such as administrative bloat and price opacity. Still, this model aligns with American values of choice and gradualism, making it a politically feasible compromise.

The most transformative, albeit contentious, scenario involves a shift toward universal care, either through single-payer systems or other mechanisms that guarantee comprehensive coverage for all. Advocates point to the moral imperative of health equity and the long-term cost savings associated with preventive care and reduced administrative complexity. This vision, however, faces formidable obstacles, including political resistance, the powerful lobbying efforts of the healthcare industry, and the cultural aversion to perceived government overreach. Transitioning to a universal system would also require significant upfront investment and a recalibration of the workforce to meet expanded demand, challenges that would test the political will and logistical capacity of policymakers.

Complicating these scenarios are external pressures, such as demographic shifts, technological advancements, and the rising prevalence of chronic diseases. An aging population will place increasing strain on Medicare and Medicaid, necessitating innovative funding solutions and care delivery models. Similarly, the integration of artificial intelligence, telemedicine, and personalized medicine offers both opportunities and risks. While these technologies promise to enhance efficiency and outcomes, they could also widen disparities if access to such advancements remains uneven.

Global health trends and economic pressures further influence the direction of U.S. healthcare. The COVID-19 pandemic underscored the interconnectedness of healthcare systems and the vulnerability of even advanced nations to public health crises. In a globalized world, U.S. policymakers must consider how trade policies, international collaborations, and the global pharmaceutical supply chain shape domestic healthcare outcomes. Economic volatility, meanwhile, may amplify calls for reform as rising costs become unsustainable for households, employers, and governments alike.

Ultimately, navigating these crossroads requires confronting fundamental questions about the purpose and values of healthcare in America. Should it remain a market-driven enterprise, or should it be treated as a public good? How can innovation coexist with equity, and how do we balance individual responsibility with collective well-being? The answers will determine not only the future of the U.S. healthcare system but also the broader social contract between the state and its citizens.

As the nation grapples with these choices, the need for bold yet pragmatic leadership is paramount. Policymakers must balance immediate needs with long-term vision, resisting the temptation to prioritize short-term gains over sustainable progress. Public engagement will also play a crucial role, as cultural narratives about healthcare's role in society evolve. Whether through grassroots advocacy, bipartisan collaboration, or disruptive innovation, the path forward will reflect the values and priorities of a nation at a pivotal moment in its history. The question is not merely what kind of healthcare system America wants, but what kind of society it aspires to be.

Chapter 12: The Global Lens – Lessons from Other Countries

The U.S. healthcare system stands as a global anomaly, its design deeply rooted in the principles of market capitalism and individualism. To understand its unique trajectory, it is instructive to examine alternative approaches in other nations—models that have evolved in response to different historical, cultural, and economic imperatives. European nations such as Germany and the United Kingdom, Canada's single-payer system, and innovative hybrid frameworks in Asia, particularly Japan and Singapore, offer instructive contrasts. These systems embody varying balances of public and private involvement, with differing priorities in cost containment, accessibility, and equity. However, the task of translating these approaches into an American context is fraught with challenges. The political, cultural, and economic fabric of the U.S. resists wholesale adoption of foreign models, reflecting profound differences in values and governance structures.

At first glance, the European experience seems to offer clear lessons. Germany's Bismarck model, with its employer-based health insurance system and private delivery of care, may appear somewhat analogous to the American approach. However, its foundation rests on principles of social solidarity and state oversight, enabling it to deliver near-universal coverage while maintaining cost control through negotiated pricing. Similarly, the United Kingdom's National Health Service (NHS), a publicly funded and administered system, exemplifies the ideal of healthcare as a social right. It provides universal, free-at-point-of-service care and achieves remarkable cost efficiency relative to other high-income countries. Yet, both models face significant pressures, from aging populations to debates about the sustainability of public funding. For the United States, these challenges underscore the complexities of adapting systems born of very different political and cultural climates. The entrenched American skepticism of state-managed programs, coupled with its deeply privatized healthcare industry, complicates any attempt to emulate European solutions.

Canada offers another point of comparison, often invoked in American debates as a nearby example of a single-payer system. The Canadian healthcare framework, shaped by mid-20th century reforms, delivers universal coverage through tax-funded provincial plans. Unlike the NHS, Canada's system separates financing from delivery, with most care provided through private practices. Administrative simplicity and equitable access are hallmarks of this approach, but it is not without flaws. Wait times for non-urgent procedures and disparities in rural versus urban care remain persistent concerns. American critics frequently seize on these shortcomings to dismiss the viability of single-payer models. However, such criticisms often ignore the broader benefits of a system that insulates individuals from the financial devastation of medical crises. At the same time, the challenges of scaling such a system to the U.S.'s vast and diverse population, coupled with the political power of private insurers, make it a difficult proposition.

Asian nations offer a different set of insights, blending elements of public oversight with market mechanisms. Japan's healthcare system, rooted in universal insurance and strict cost regulation, achieves some of the best health outcomes in the world. It emphasizes preventive care and cost control, with the government negotiating prices to ensure affordability. Similarly, Singapore has developed an innovative framework that combines mandatory savings accounts, government subsidies, and private insurance. This system incentivizes individual responsibility for healthcare costs while ensuring a safety net for those unable to pay. These models, however, operate within socio-economic and cultural contexts that prioritize communal welfare and high levels of trust in government—a stark contrast to the American emphasis on personal autonomy and mistrust of centralized authority. Moreover, the scale and demographic pressures of the U.S. further complicate the feasibility of replicating such approaches.

Ultimately, the obstacles to importing foreign healthcare models into the U.S. extend beyond logistical considerations. At their core, these challenges reflect fundamental differences in values and governance. European and Asian systems largely treat healthcare as a public good, underpinned by collective responsibility. The American system, by contrast, views healthcare as both a commodity and a personal responsibility, a perspective shaped by the nation's broader commitment to free-market principles. This divergence is reinforced by a political landscape deeply resistant to sweeping reforms, with powerful lobbying groups and fragmented federal-state dynamics further entrenching the status quo. Efforts to implement systemic change must therefore contend not only with structural inertia but also with cultural and ideological barriers.

Comparisons with other nations highlight both the possibilities and the limitations of reform. While the U.S. can draw valuable lessons from global practices—whether in cost regulation, preventative care, or universal access—such insights must be tailored to its unique context. The challenge lies in identifying pragmatic, incremental changes that align with American values while addressing the inequities and inefficiencies that persist. A wholesale adoption of foreign models is unlikely, but selective integration of their principles offers a path toward a more equitable and sustainable healthcare system.

Europe's Social Insurance Models

Europe's social insurance models offer a nuanced perspective on healthcare systems built around the principles of solidarity, equity, and collective responsibility. These models, while varying across nations, share a foundational commitment to ensuring universal access to healthcare through mechanisms that balance public oversight with private sector involvement. Germany's Bismarck model, established in the late 19th century, exemplifies this approach. Its framework is centered on employer-based health insurance, with contributions shared between employers and employees. The system is characterized by decentralized administration, with numerous sickness funds operating under strict government regulation to ensure standardization and fairness. While the delivery of care remains largely privatized, Germany's model achieves cost containment and broad access through negotiated pricing and mandatory participation.

This balance between public oversight and private autonomy is further evident in France's healthcare system, which builds on similar principles. Like Germany, France relies on a system of social insurance, with healthcare financing derived from payroll taxes and supplemented by government contributions. However, the French model incorporates a higher degree of state involvement, particularly in regulating fees and reimbursing citizens for medical expenses. Patients maintain the freedom to choose their providers, fostering competition and efficiency, while the government ensures that out-of-pocket expenses remain minimal. Both systems exemplify how social insurance models can blend market dynamics with a robust safety net, creating a framework that prioritizes both individual choice and collective welfare.

A notable feature of these models is their ability to deliver high-quality care at a fraction of the per capita cost of the U.S. system. Administrative efficiency, achieved through standardized billing practices and universal participation, plays a critical role in reducing overhead expenses. Moreover, the emphasis on negotiated pricing between insurers and providers ensures that costs remain transparent and controlled. This approach stands in stark contrast to the fragmented, opaque pricing mechanisms that characterize American healthcare. While proponents of U.S. reform often cite these efficiencies as evidence of the superiority of social insurance models, significant cultural and structural differences complicate their direct transplantation to the American context.

Despite their successes, Europe's social insurance models face challenges that underscore the complexities of universal coverage. Aging populations and rising healthcare demands have strained financial resources, prompting debates about sustainability and reform. Germany, for instance, has introduced measures to cap costs, such as reducing reimbursement rates and encouraging generic drug use. In France, efforts to balance quality and cost have led to incremental changes in reimbursement policies and an increased emphasis on preventative care. These challenges illustrate that no system is immune to pressures from demographic shifts and technological advances. They also serve as a reminder that the adaptability of social insurance systems is crucial to their continued success.

For the United States, the appeal of Europe's social insurance models lies in their ability to reconcile universal access with the preservation of private sector roles. However, such systems operate within cultural frameworks that differ fundamentally from American values. European nations generally exhibit a greater degree of trust in government institutions and a stronger collective ethos, which underpin public acceptance of mandatory participation and income-based contributions. In contrast, the U.S. healthcare system reflects an individualistic culture that prioritizes personal choice and skepticism of centralized control. Efforts to adapt elements of the Bismarck model, for example, would face significant resistance from both political stakeholders and segments of the population wary of perceived government overreach.

Europe's social insurance models provide valuable lessons in achieving equity, efficiency, and quality through a balanced approach. However, their potential applicability to the U.S. context lies not in wholesale adoption but in selective adaptation. Elements such as standardized billing practices, negotiated pricing, and an emphasis on preventative care could inform American reforms, offering pathways to address some of the systemic inefficiencies and disparities that persist. Yet, any such efforts must account for the unique cultural, political, and economic realities that shape the American healthcare landscape, emphasizing pragmatic solutions over idealistic aspirations.

CANADA'S SINGLE-PAYER SYSTEM

Canada's single-payer healthcare system offers an alternative lens through which to examine the possibilities and limitations of universal coverage. Widely regarded as one of the most straightforward and equitable healthcare models, Canada's approach rests on the foundational principles of universality, accessibility, portability, comprehensiveness, and public administration—values enshrined in the Canada Health Act of 1984. Under this framework, the government serves as the sole payer for medically necessary services, funded primarily through general taxation. By eliminating private insurers for essential healthcare, Canada has successfully reduced administrative costs and ensured that all citizens, regardless of income or employment status, have access to a standardized level of care.

At its core, Canada's system decentralizes healthcare administration, with each province and territory responsible for designing and managing its healthcare delivery in accordance with federal guidelines. This provincial autonomy allows for flexibility in meeting local needs while maintaining a uniform commitment to universal coverage. Unlike the multi-payer system in the United States, Canada's single-payer model eliminates the complexity of competing insurance plans, streamlining patient access to care and reducing inefficiencies tied to billing and reimbursement. Hospitals receive annual budgets, and physicians are paid on a fee-for-service basis, with reimbursement rates negotiated between provincial health authorities and medical associations. This simplicity has translated into remarkable cost control, with Canada spending approximately half as much per capita on healthcare as the United States, despite achieving comparable health outcomes in key areas.

However, Canada's system is not without its limitations, which are often cited as cautionary tales in debates about adopting a single-payer approach in the

United States. Chief among these challenges is the issue of wait times for non-urgent procedures and specialist care. The budgetary constraints that enable cost containment also place limitations on resource availability, creating bottlenecks in certain areas of the system. While emergency and primary care remain accessible without significant delays, patients seeking elective surgeries, diagnostic imaging, or specialist consultations often face longer wait periods. Critics argue that these delays reflect inefficiencies inherent to a publicly funded system, though proponents counter that they are the trade-offs of prioritizing equity over immediate access for a privileged few.

The Canadian experience also highlights the tension between universality and privatization. While the public system covers medically necessary services, it does not extend to pharmaceuticals, dental care, or vision services, which are often financed through private insurance or out-of-pocket payments. This creates a secondary tier of healthcare access that disproportionately affects lower-income Canadians, underscoring the ongoing challenges of addressing gaps within a single-payer framework. Recent debates about introducing more private sector involvement to alleviate pressures on the public system further reveal the delicate balance between preserving equity and responding to rising demands.

From the American perspective, Canada's single-payer system holds both promise and provocation. Advocates of single-payer healthcare in the United States often cite Canada as a model for achieving universality without significantly increasing overall costs. The simplicity of the system—its ability to pool risk, streamline administration, and negotiate prices—offers an attractive counterpoint to the fragmented, profit-driven nature of American healthcare. By consolidating purchasing power under a single public entity, Canada has demonstrated the feasibility of negotiating lower drug prices and service costs, a strategy that could mitigate the exorbitant expenditures that burden the U.S. system.

Yet, the cultural and structural differences between Canada and the United States complicate any direct application of the Canadian model. Canada's system operates within a context of societal trust in public institutions and an acceptance of healthcare as a collective right. The United States, by contrast, grapples with deep-rooted skepticism toward government intervention and a preference for individual choice and market-based solutions. Efforts to establish single-payer healthcare in the U.S., such as proposals for "Medicare for All," have faced fierce resistance, driven by ideological opposition, concerns over increased taxation, and the influence of powerful stakeholders in the insurance and pharmaceutical industries.

Moreover, Canada's relative homogeneity and smaller population simplify the administration of its healthcare system in ways that would be difficult to replicate in a diverse, highly decentralized nation like the United States. The American healthcare landscape, shaped by a long history of employer-based insurance and private sector dominance, presents structural barriers to the transition toward a publicly financed model. Resistance from entrenched interests, coupled with fears of long wait times and perceived reductions in quality, further complicate the political feasibility of adopting a Canadian-style system.

Ultimately, Canada's single-payer experience offers valuable insights into the benefits and trade-offs of prioritizing equity and cost control within a public framework. While the U.S. can draw lessons from Canada's successes—particularly in areas like administrative simplification, cost negotiation, and universal primary care access—any effort to adapt such a model must address the unique cultural, economic, and political realities that define American society. The Canadian system is not a panacea, but it serves as a compelling case study for reimagining healthcare as a public good rather than a market commodity, challenging Americans to reconsider the values that underpin their own system.

Asia's Emerging Hybrid Models

Asia's emerging hybrid models present a fascinating convergence of public commitment to healthcare equity and private sector dynamism, offering nuanced solutions that reflect the region's rapid economic development, demographic pressures, and diverse cultural contexts. Across countries such as Japan, South Korea, China, and Singapore, healthcare systems balance universal access with market-driven efficiencies, blending elements of social insurance, government subsidies, and private enterprise. These systems demonstrate that achieving broad coverage and cost control does not necessarily require the wholesale rejection of capitalist principles but rather a strategic synthesis of public oversight and private innovation. For the United States, Asia's experience offers valuable lessons on adaptability, pragmatism, and the importance of context-specific design.

In Japan and South Korea, two of the most advanced economies in Asia, the foundation of healthcare rests on compulsory social insurance systems that ensure universal coverage while incorporating private-sector participation. Japan's healthcare model, established after World War II, operates on a multi-payer system where citizens are required to enroll in public insurance programs tied either to employment or residence. The system emphasizes affordability, with strict government control over medical fees, uniform reimbursement rates, and robust price negotiations that curtail excessive costs. Patients enjoy freedom of choice in selecting doctors and facilities, with private providers delivering the majority of healthcare services within the public insurance framework. South Korea adopts a similarly structured National Health Insurance (NHI) system, achieving near-universal coverage by pooling contributions from employees, employers, and government subsidies. These models demonstrate how market incentives, such as competition among providers, can coexist with strong state regulation to ensure access, efficiency, and quality.

However, challenges remain. Both Japan and South Korea grapple with aging populations that place immense pressure on healthcare resources and costs. In Japan, where nearly 30% of the population is over 65, the rising demand for chronic care, long-term care services, and technological advancements stretches the system's financial sustainability. Meanwhile, South Korea's healthcare providers often rely on private payments for uncovered services, creating concerns about growing disparities in access. Nonetheless, these systems exemplify how combining public financing with private delivery—while rigorously regulating costs—can achieve equitable outcomes without compromising individual choice.

China, as the world's most populous country, offers a different narrative: one of dramatic transformation in pursuit of accessible healthcare for all. Historically, China's healthcare system suffered from underinvestment following market reforms in the 1980s, which led to a reliance on out-of-pocket payments and vast rural-urban inequalities. Over the past two decades, however, China has embarked on ambitious reforms to achieve near-universal coverage through public insurance schemes supported by significant government investment. Rural and urban residents are now covered by distinct insurance programs, while the state heavily subsidizes care for vulnerable populations. Simultaneously, China embraces private sector participation to expand service delivery and improve innovation, especially in urban areas. The country's success in mobilizing resources to extend basic coverage to over 95% of its population is a testament to the role of political will and state capacity in driving healthcare reform. Yet, challenges persist, particularly in ensuring equitable access between rural and urban regions and curbing rising costs tied to an overreliance on out-of-pocket expenditures for pharmaceuticals and specialized care.

Singapore represents one of the most intriguing hybrid models, blending rigorous state control with market mechanisms to create a system that is efficient, equitable, and cost-conscious. Singapore's healthcare model is built upon the principle of shared responsibility between the government, individuals, and employers, underpinned by the "3M" framework: MediSave, MediShield, and MediFund. MediSave, a mandatory health savings account, requires individuals to set aside a portion of their wages to cover personal and family medical expenses. MediShield, a low-cost insurance program, provides catastrophic coverage for major illnesses, while MediFund serves as a safety net for low-income citizens who cannot afford care. This tiered system ensures that individuals take financial responsibility for routine expenses while the state intervenes to protect against catastrophic risks. The result is a system that achieves excellent health outcomes—Singapore consistently ranks among the healthiest nations globally—while keeping healthcare spending below 5% of GDP, a fraction of U.S. expenditure.

Critics of the Singapore model note that its emphasis on individual responsibility may not easily translate to larger, more heterogeneous societies like the United States. While Singapore's small size, centralized governance, and culturally cohesive population enable seamless implementation, scaling such a system to a country as vast and diverse as the United States poses immense logistical and political challenges. Additionally, Singapore's healthcare culture places strong emphasis on personal savings and thrift, reflecting societal norms that may be difficult to replicate in a more consumption-oriented American context.

Asia's emerging healthcare models collectively illustrate the importance of pragmatism and adaptability in designing systems that reflect economic, cultural, and demographic realities. These countries demonstrate that universal access need not entail a rigid rejection of market principles; rather, it requires deliberate regulation, shared financial responsibility, and strategic public-private partnerships. For the United States, where ideological divides often stall healthcare reform, Asia's experience underscores the value of incremental, context-specific solutions over sweeping overhauls. The Asian models also challenge the American tendency to equate privatization with efficiency, revealing that strong state oversight—when paired with market incentives—can produce outcomes that balance access, quality, and cost.

Yet, the cultural and structural barriers to implementing similar approaches in the United States remain considerable. While Japan, South Korea, China, and Singapore operate within frameworks of collective responsibility and state legitimacy, the United States continues to prioritize individual autonomy and market freedom. Bridging these ideological divides requires not just policy innovation but a broader cultural shift in how healthcare is perceived—as both a personal responsibility and a societal good. Asia's hybrid models, with their capacity for balance and adaptability, offer valuable lessons for an American system that remains burdened by inefficiencies, inequities, and runaway costs. The challenge lies not in replicating these models wholesale but in extracting principles that can inform a uniquely American approach to healthcare reform.

WHY IMPORTING MODELS IS DIFFICULT

Importing foreign healthcare models into the United States, even when they demonstrate efficiency, equity, and lower costs, has proven an almost insurmountable challenge due to a combination of cultural, political, economic, and structural factors. At the heart of this resistance lies a fundamental tension between the values underpinning successful healthcare systems abroad and those deeply embedded in American society. While many countries prioritize collective responsibility and view healthcare as a universal right, the United States operates within an ideological framework that emphasizes individual autonomy, limited government intervention, and the primacy of market forces. These differences are not merely academic or rhetorical—they are woven into the nation's historical development, policy debates, and the expectations of its citizens, making the wholesale adoption of foreign systems impractical, if not impossible.

Cultural values form the first and most significant barrier to importing foreign healthcare models. In countries such as Japan, Canada, and much of Europe, healthcare is viewed as a shared social good, a reflection of collective responsibility for citizens' well-being. The success of systems like Canada's single-payer model or Japan's universal insurance rests on a cultural consensus that access to healthcare should be equitable and not determined by one's ability to pay. In contrast, American cultural attitudes toward healthcare reflect the country's broader ethos of rugged individualism. Healthcare is often framed as a commodity, a service that individuals must earn or purchase based on personal effort and financial resources. This cultural lens underpins resistance to universal healthcare proposals, which many Americans perceive as antithetical to their notions of freedom and choice. Efforts to position healthcare as a right are often derided as "socialist" and incompatible with the nation's capitalist ideals.

This cultural resistance is further reinforced by the entrenched political and economic interests that shape the American healthcare system. Unlike many European and Asian countries that reformed their systems at times of societal upheaval or under strong centralized leadership, the United States has seen healthcare policy evolve incrementally, with powerful private stakeholders firmly embedded in the system. Insurance companies, pharmaceutical corporations, hospital networks, and healthcare lobbyists hold immense influence over legislative processes, investing billions to protect their interests. Attempts to overhaul the system, such as efforts to establish a single-payer model or expand government-run programs, have been consistently derailed by these stakeholders, who frame reforms as threats to economic freedom, job creation, and innovation. For instance, the Affordable Care Act, despite being a relatively moderate reform, faced vehement opposition and remains a polarizing issue. The financial and political power of private industry creates a formidable barrier to importing models that prioritize state control and cost regulation, as seen in countries like Singapore or France.

Economics also play a critical role in the difficulty of implementing foreign healthcare systems in the United States. While European and Asian countries achieve universal or near-universal coverage through varying levels of public funding and cost regulation, the U.S. healthcare system is built upon a fragmented, market-driven foundation that incentivizes profit maximization. This fragmentation has resulted in the highest healthcare spending per capita globally, yet with significant disparities in access and outcomes. The entrenched nature of employer-based insurance—originating in post-World War II labor practices—has tied healthcare coverage to employment, creating a unique economic dynamic that is absent in most other countries. Proposals to decouple healthcare from employment or transition to public insurance models face immense resistance from businesses and unions alike, as such changes would disrupt existing financial arrangements, benefits structures, and labor negotiations. The economic inertia of a system so deeply tied to private markets makes the wholesale importation of centralized models, like Canada's or the UK's National Health Service, logistically and politically untenable.

Structural barriers also hinder the feasibility of adopting foreign models. The United States is a geographically vast, demographically diverse, and administratively decentralized nation. Healthcare systems in countries like Canada or South Korea succeed, in part, because they operate within more centralized governance frameworks and serve populations with greater cultural homogeneity. In contrast, the United States' federal structure, with significant power devolved to individual states, creates disparities in how healthcare is delivered, funded, and regulated. Attempts to impose a uniform national system inevitably clash with states' rights and local governance priorities, as seen in the patchwork implementation of Medicaid expansion under the Affordable Care Act. Moreover, the demographic diversity of the U.S.—with its varying healthcare needs across rural, urban, immigrant, and socioeconomically diverse populations—complicates efforts to replicate models designed for smaller, more uniform societies.

Beyond these practical barriers, there is also a fundamental question of political will. Many of the successful healthcare systems in Europe, Canada, and Asia emerged from moments of collective resolve to address societal inequities, often in the wake of war, economic collapse, or widespread public demand for reform. In contrast, the United States' political landscape is deeply polarized, with healthcare reform serving as a perennial flashpoint for ideological battles rather than a unifying cause. The cycles of healthcare debates—characterized by sweeping proposals, fierce resistance, and watered-down compromises—underscore the difficulty of achieving consensus on a path forward. While other nations have demonstrated that universal coverage and cost containment can coexist with quality care, the United States remains mired in debates over whether healthcare should be a public good at all.

Despite these challenges, the difficulty of importing foreign models does not negate the relevance of lessons that can be drawn from other countries. The principles underpinning successful systems abroad—cost control through regulation, shared financial responsibility, investment in preventive care, and the integration of public and private sectors—hold significant value for American healthcare reform. However, these principles must be adapted rather than adopted wholesale, tailored to align with the United States' unique cultural, economic, and political realities. Achieving meaningful reform requires bridging the ideological divides that have long defined the American approach to healthcare, fostering a cultural shift that balances individual choice with collective responsibility. While importing foreign models may be infeasible, extracting their most effective components offers a pragmatic path forward—one that acknowledges the strengths of the U.S. system while addressing its profound inefficiencies and inequities.

Lessons for the U.S.

While importing foreign healthcare models wholesale remains a practical and cultural impossibility for the United States, there are critical lessons to be gleaned from systems abroad. These insights provide a pathway to incremental reforms that align with American values while addressing the systemic inefficiencies, inequities, and exorbitant costs that define the U.S. healthcare landscape. By identifying and adapting the most effective principles of care delivery, cost containment, and patient outcomes, the United States can move toward a healthcare system that works for a broader population without abandoning its foundational ideals of choice, innovation, and market-driven efficiency.

First and foremost, the lesson of cost control through regulation emerges as a consistent feature of successful healthcare systems worldwide. Countries like France, Germany, and Japan have shown that rigorous price negotiation and rate-setting—whether for drugs, hospital services, or provider fees—can keep healthcare spending in check without sacrificing quality. These nations employ a combination of government oversight and public-private partnerships to ensure fair pricing across the healthcare value chain. For instance, Japan's fee schedule, updated regularly to balance provider sustainability with affordability, demonstrates that market forces can coexist with state-led regulation to contain costs. In contrast, the United States' largely unregulated pricing mechanisms have created runaway costs, driven by opaque negotiations, monopolistic practices, and profit incentives. Adopting targeted price controls for pharmaceuticals, medical devices, and insurance reimbursements would not dismantle the American market economy but would curb the system's inefficiencies.

Second, the United States can learn from the principle of universal access, not as a rigid single-payer system but as a moral and economic imperative. Countries with vastly different economic and political contexts—such as Canada's single-payer system, Germany's multi-payer model, and Singapore's hybrid structure—demonstrate that healthcare can be treated as a right while leveraging market incentives. The lesson is not in the specific architecture of these systems but in their shared commitment to ensuring baseline coverage for all citizens. Universal access reduces long-term costs by improving preventive care, minimizing expensive emergency interventions, and ensuring that individuals receive treatment before their health conditions escalate. For the United States, this principle need not imply the elimination of private insurance or choice; instead, it could manifest in an expanded public option or hybrid system where baseline coverage is guaranteed, and supplemental private options coexist.

Another critical lesson lies in the prioritization of preventive care and primary care services, a hallmark of effective healthcare systems across Europe and Asia. Countries like Denmark and South Korea have invested heavily in robust primary care networks that act as gatekeepers to specialty services. This focus ensures that patients receive timely, cost-effective care while avoiding unnecessary procedures and hospitalizations. In contrast, the U.S. healthcare system's over-reliance on specialist care and its fragmented delivery structure drive up costs and produce inconsistent outcomes. Strengthening primary care infrastructure in the United States—through financial incentives for family physicians, telemedicine expansion, and community-based care models—would improve population health while reducing the economic burden on hospitals and patients.

Furthermore, the integration of public and private sectors, as seen in countries like Germany and Singapore, offers valuable lessons for the U.S. healthcare system. Germany's multi-payer model demonstrates that competition among private insurers can be structured to prioritize patient welfare when operating within a tightly regulated framework. Similarly, Singapore's hybrid approach combines individual responsibility, government subsidies, and market-driven efficiencies to balance affordability with quality. These systems illustrate that universal access need not preclude innovation, competition, or individual choice—values that resonate deeply with American ideals. For the United States, the lesson is clear: the government and private sector can collaborate to build a more equitable and efficient system without relinquishing market dynamics entirely.

Lessons from other countries also highlight the importance of addressing social determinants of health—factors like housing, education, nutrition, and income inequality—that directly influence health outcomes. Nations with successful healthcare systems recognize that medical care alone cannot improve population health; broader social policies must work in tandem with healthcare delivery. For instance, Nordic countries invest heavily in social programs that reduce poverty and improve living conditions, leading to better overall health and lower healthcare expenditures. While the United States faces unique challenges in addressing social determinants due to its size, diversity, and political resistance to welfare spending, targeted investments in public health initiatives—such as nutrition programs, mental health services, and housing support—would yield significant long-term benefits.

Additionally, the emphasis on transparency and accountability in healthcare systems abroad offers another critical lesson. Countries like the United Kingdom and Japan have implemented systems that ensure clear communication of costs, quality metrics, and outcomes to patients and providers alike. This transparency fosters trust, reduces unnecessary spending, and empowers individuals to make informed decisions about their care. In the United States, where opaque billing practices and complex insurance structures often leave patients confused and vulnerable to medical debt, greater transparency—through standardized pricing, simplified billing, and public reporting of provider performance—would improve both the efficiency and fairness of the system.

Finally, global models underscore the importance of political consensus and public engagement in achieving meaningful healthcare reform. Successful systems abroad emerged not merely from technical solutions but from collective societal resolve to prioritize health as a shared value. While the United States remains deeply divided on the role of government in healthcare, fostering bipartisan dialogue and engaging the public in conversations about the trade-offs of reform are critical steps toward change. Other nations demonstrate that healthcare systems can evolve through incremental reforms, provided there is a shared understanding of the system's goals.

In adapting these lessons, the United States need not abandon its unique identity or foundational values. The goal is not to import an external blueprint but to extract the most effective principles and tailor them to the American context. By embracing cost control, universal access, preventive care, public-private collaboration, and transparency, the United States can move toward a system that balances equity, innovation, and sustainability. The challenge lies in reconciling these lessons with the deeply held cultural, political, and economic forces that define American healthcare. While no single foreign model will ever perfectly fit the United States, the cumulative wisdom of other nations offers a roadmap for progress—one that honors the complexities of the U.S. system while striving for a more just and efficient future.

NO ONE-SIZE-FITS-ALL SOLUTION

At the heart of global comparisons lies a profound recognition: no single healthcare system, no matter how successful in its home country, can serve as a universal template for others. Healthcare is not a static construct; it is a product of history, politics, economics, and culture, each uniquely shaping the systems that exist today. Attempting to impose a one-size-fits-all solution ignores the deep contextual roots that make a system function in its specific environment. The United States, with its unique blend of individualism, market orientation, and political fragmentation, underscores this reality more starkly than most. Its challenges cannot be met with a wholesale adoption of European, Canadian, or Asian models; they require solutions tailored to America's values, constraints, and deeply ingrained social dynamics.

In Europe, social solidarity and collectivism undergird healthcare systems that prioritize equity and universal access. For many European nations, the notion of healthcare as a collective right is not up for debate but is instead woven into the fabric of societal expectations. This philosophical alignment enables public buy-in for taxation structures that fund healthcare systems and for regulatory measures that control costs. In contrast, the United States' individualistic ethos—where autonomy, choice, and self-determination reign—creates resistance to policies perceived as paternalistic or redistributive. The political appetite for higher taxes to fund universal coverage remains limited, and the cultural preference for individualized solutions often supersedes collective approaches. The European systems work because they align with the cultural norms of their populations; for the United States, adopting such models wholesale would disregard a foundational pillar of American identity.

Canada's single-payer system further highlights the importance of historical and institutional context. The Canadian model emerged as part of a postwar national movement toward equality and access, deeply rooted in federal-provincial collaboration and public consensus. However, Canada's smaller population, provincial-level administration, and relatively homogenous political values provided fertile ground for single-payer healthcare to take hold. The United States, in contrast, faces significant structural obstacles, including its size, diversity, and decentralized governance. A single-payer system would require not only a massive overhaul of existing infrastructure but also the resolution of contentious federal-state power dynamics. Moreover, implementing such a model in the U.S. would require addressing the entrenched influence of private insurers, pharmaceutical companies, and hospital networks—actors with vested interests in maintaining the status quo. Canada's system cannot simply be "transplanted" into an American context without triggering enormous political, economic, and cultural upheaval.

Asia's emerging hybrid models offer a different lesson: pragmatism and adaptability. Countries like Singapore, South Korea, and Japan demonstrate that systems can be designed to balance market efficiency with government oversight. Yet these successes are predicated on unique political and cultural conditions that cannot be easily replicated. Singapore's mandatory savings accounts, for instance, depend on a strong culture of government trust and individual responsibility, reinforced by decades of effective state planning. South Korea's rapid development of its single-payer model reflects a cultural emphasis on collective progress and national development, combined with a relatively young, healthy population at the time of implementation. These conditions are markedly different from the United States, where skepticism toward government involvement remains high, and a large, aging population places significant strain on any proposed reforms. The adaptability seen in Asian models is instructive, but their success cannot be divorced from their local contexts.

Beyond the cultural and political dimensions, economic realities further underscore the difficulty of universal solutions. In many nations with highly effective healthcare systems, cost containment has been achieved through regulatory measures, government bargaining power, and limited profit incentives. The United States, however, operates within a deeply market-driven framework where healthcare is not just a service but a massive industry generating trillions of dollars annually. The intertwining of healthcare with employment, private insurance markets, and investor-driven hospitals creates an economic dependency that resists fundamental change. Transitioning to a model that reduces profits for powerful stakeholders would necessitate overcoming significant political resistance and addressing concerns about job loss, economic disruption, and innovation. No country with a successful healthcare system contends with a for-profit structure as deeply entrenched as the one in the United States.

The diversity of healthcare systems around the world serves as a reminder that there are multiple pathways to achieving health equity, access, and cost efficiency. While the principles of universal access, cost control, and preventive care can be found in nearly all successful models, their implementation must be adapted to fit local contexts. For the United States, this means acknowledging its unique challenges while extracting the most relevant lessons from abroad. Incremental reforms, such as expanding public options, controlling pharmaceutical prices, or enhancing primary care infrastructure, are far more realistic than a wholesale shift to a foreign model. These reforms can align with American values of choice, innovation, and market competition while addressing the most glaring inefficiencies and inequities in the system.

Ultimately, the search for a single "perfect" healthcare system is misguided. Every system reflects the priorities and compromises of the society it serves. In the United States, where healthcare is both a moral issue and a deeply embedded industry, the path forward requires balancing innovation with regulation, individual choice with collective responsibility, and short-term pragmatism with long-term vision. While no external model can be imported in its entirety, the cumulative lessons from other countries offer a blueprint for building a healthcare system that is uniquely American—one that reflects the nation's values while striving to correct its failures. The challenge is not to replicate what works elsewhere but to adapt those principles to an American framework, forging a system that serves both the ideals and practical realities of the United States.

CHAPTER 13: HEALTHCARE THAT WORKS – WITHOUT BREAKING THE SYSTEM

The narrative surrounding capitalism and healthcare is often reduced to a binary argument: either the market serves as an engine of innovation or a barrier to equitable care. This oversimplification conceals the nuances of how market principles can be realigned to work in favor of both access and efficiency without fundamentally altering the economic foundation. The U.S. healthcare system, deeply embedded in capitalist logic, has not failed because of capitalism itself but because it has allowed distortions to corrode the mechanisms of competition. Instead of leveraging the system's inherent strengths—its ability to foster innovation, reward efficiency, and drive progress—healthcare in America has permitted monopolistic practices, opaque cost structures, and incentives detached from patient outcomes to define its trajectory. Capitalism, when properly constrained and strategically recalibrated, does not inherently conflict with the principles of care; rather, it offers an opportunity to reshape healthcare as a dynamic, value-driven ecosystem where profitability aligns with patient well-being.

What has emerged in the United States is a market distorted by unchecked consolidation, where large insurers, pharmaceutical companies, and provider networks have neutralized the competitive forces that should be lowering costs and improving outcomes. Monopolies have grown under the guise of efficiency, yet their effect has been to narrow options, inflate prices, and leave patients powerless. Meanwhile, the hidden nature of healthcare costs—where pricing is cloaked in a fog of ambiguity—prevents consumers from making informed choices, undermining a core tenet of capitalism: transparency. Patients, now stripped of their agency, navigate a system in which economic logic has been applied selectively, favoring profit-maximization without accountability.

The misalignment of incentives compounds this dysfunction. The dominance of fee-for-service models, which reward providers based on volume rather than value, has entrenched inefficiency and overtreatment while sidelining preventive care. Healthcare professionals operate within structures that prioritize billing codes over patient outcomes, perpetuating a cycle where financial success does not equate to better health. The system itself incentivizes fragmentation—disconnected services, overlapping procedures, and administrative bloat—while neglecting the long-term investments required to keep populations healthier and costs lower. Capitalism, left unshaped by thoughtful regulation, has drifted from its promise of delivering value through competition.

Redefining the role of capitalism in healthcare begins with recognizing that market principles can be a force for systemic reform if directed toward correcting these distortions. The solution does not lie in dismantling the market but in reintroducing the forces it requires to thrive: competition, transparency, and value-based incentives. This is not a rejection of capitalism but its restoration to purpose. Innovation, one of the market's most powerful tools, must be encouraged not merely in the development of costly treatments but in the design of delivery systems, payment models, and technologies that prioritize accessibility and efficiency. Competition must be actively nurtured through anti-trust enforcement, ensuring that no single entity—whether insurer, pharmaceutical company, or hospital network—can dominate the market and stifle its dynamism. Pricing transparency must shift from being an abstract ideal to a functional standard, empowering patients to understand and choose between options, driving costs downward through informed demand.

There is nothing inherently incompatible between capitalism and the provision of equitable, effective care. To argue otherwise is to deny the potential for a market-driven system that rewards outcomes rather than volume, efficiency rather than exploitation. Redefining capitalism's role in healthcare means moving beyond ideological constraints and acknowledging that the system can evolve to serve the public good while preserving its economic foundations. It requires pragmatic, deliberate reform that channels market energy toward innovation, affordability, and accountability. By aligning profit with patient well-being, healthcare in America can escape its current contradictions and fulfill its unkept promise: a system where competition drives quality, access expands without disruption, and the market works for those it was designed to serve.

WHERE THE MARKET FAILS: IDENTIFYING SYSTEMIC INEFFICIENCIES

While capitalism has the potential to drive efficiency, innovation, and improved outcomes, its application within the U.S. healthcare system reveals critical failures that exacerbate systemic inefficiencies. These failures are not inherent to market principles but result from a confluence of misaligned incentives, insufficient regulation, and the dominance of entrenched interests that exploit the system's complexity. What should function as a competitive marketplace, where value and quality drive success, has instead evolved into a fragmented ecosystem where inefficiencies thrive unchecked, costs balloon, and patients are left underserved.

At its core, healthcare in America suffers from a fundamental misalignment between the interests of providers, insurers, pharmaceutical companies, and patients. In a truly functional market, providers would compete to deliver the highest quality care at the lowest possible cost. Instead, the dominance of fee-for-service reimbursement has turned healthcare into a volume-driven enterprise where more procedures, tests, and treatments are rewarded regardless of their necessity or impact on patient outcomes. This creates a system in which overtreatment becomes not an anomaly but a structural inevitability, bloating costs while delivering diminishing returns in population health.

Insurance markets further expose the inefficiencies of the current structure. While competition in theory should drive down premiums and expand coverage options, the consolidation of insurers has resulted in reduced competition and monopolistic control. Large players dictate terms to both providers and patients, imposing bureaucratic hurdles that prioritize administrative cost-saving measures over care delivery. Patients are often left navigating labyrinthine networks, denied coverage for essential treatments, or burdened by out-of-pocket costs that are opaque until a bill arrives. The result is a market that functions less like a dynamic ecosystem and more like a cartelized oligopoly, where power rests in the hands of a few, and the consumer—the patient—loses both choice and leverage.

Pharmaceutical pricing offers another striking example of systemic market failure. Unlike other markets, where competition drives down costs over time, the pharmaceutical industry operates under distorted incentives that protect profits at the expense of affordability. Patent monopolies extend indefinitely through incremental modifications, generics are strategically delayed, and prices remain unshackled by any meaningful cost-control mechanisms. Drugs that are essential for survival become inaccessible luxuries, while pharmaceutical companies reap unprecedented margins. Rather than rewarding innovation that enhances public health, the market rewards price inflation and strategic exploitation of regulatory loopholes.

Administrative inefficiency compounds these structural problems. A significant portion of healthcare spending in the United States is consumed not by care itself but by the labyrinthine bureaucracy of insurance claims, coding requirements, and redundant administrative processes. Unlike other sectors, where streamlined operations reduce costs, healthcare has fostered an environment in which complexity is monetized. Hospitals and providers must employ extensive administrative staff to navigate reimbursement protocols, appeals, and billing disputes—costs ultimately passed on to patients and insurers. The result is a system where a staggering percentage of expenditures are absorbed not by care delivery but by intermediaries who add no tangible value to patient outcomes.

Systemic inefficiencies are further entrenched by the fragmentation of care delivery. Patients often receive treatment across disconnected providers, each operating in isolation with little coordination or shared accountability. This fragmentation leads to duplicative tests, gaps in care, and poor health management, particularly for chronic diseases that require integrated, long-term strategies. Preventive care, which could alleviate downstream costs and improve population health, remains woefully underemphasized because the financial incentives favor acute interventions and episodic treatments. In this distorted market, short-term profitability outweighs long-term efficiency, and patients bear the brunt of the consequences.

The failures of the U.S. healthcare market reflect a system that has allowed its own mechanisms to calcify. Rather than driving innovation and value, competition has been stifled, incentives have been warped, and inefficiencies have become embedded as structural norms. Addressing these failures does not require rejecting market principles but acknowledging their misapplication. True reform must focus on restoring competition, enforcing transparency, and aligning financial incentives with health outcomes. Systemic inefficiencies are not inevitable—they are the byproducts of a healthcare economy that has strayed from its intended purpose. By identifying these points of failure and addressing their root causes, the healthcare system can be steered toward a future where market dynamics work in service of efficiency, affordability, and patient-centered care.

Harnessing Market Forces for Reform

Harnessing market forces for reform requires a recalibration of incentives, structures, and priorities so that capitalism functions as it was originally intended: driving competition, innovation, and value while delivering meaningful benefits to patients. The current healthcare system demonstrates not the failure of market principles but the distortion of their application. If properly harnessed, these forces could transform healthcare into a more equitable, efficient, and effective system without dismantling its capitalist foundation. Reforming healthcare through market dynamics demands recognizing where the system has deviated from its purpose and designing pragmatic solutions that restore competition, reward value, and enhance consumer agency.

At the heart of this approach lies a shift from volume-based to value-based care. Rather than rewarding providers for the quantity of services performed, reforms must incentivize outcomes that matter—better health, improved quality of life, and reduced long-term costs. Value-based payment models, such as bundled payments, capitation, and shared savings programs, align provider incentives with patient well-being by tying compensation to measurable outcomes rather than sheer output. When providers are rewarded for preventing illness, managing chronic conditions effectively, and coordinating care efficiently, the system begins to prioritize health over profit. This shift does not reject capitalism but instead reorients its rewards toward performance and accountability.

Restoring genuine competition is equally critical. While healthcare markets currently suffer from consolidation and monopolistic tendencies, reforms can break down barriers to entry, expand consumer choice, and drive down costs. Policies that encourage transparency in pricing, outcomes, and quality metrics would empower patients to make informed decisions, creating a more dynamic market where providers must compete on value rather than relying on opaque pricing structures or network exclusivity. By mandating clear cost disclosures and fostering platforms where patients can compare providers, insurers, and treatment options, reform can inject the very competition that capitalism requires to thrive.

Pharmaceutical markets represent a particularly urgent area for intervention. To harness market forces effectively, the rules of engagement must change. Regulatory reforms that limit patent manipulation, promote generic competition, and allow negotiated pricing can drive down drug costs without stifling innovation. The pharmaceutical industry, when freed from its current distortions, has the potential to achieve its dual mandate: generating profits through groundbreaking treatments while maintaining access and affordability for patients. Competitive pricing structures, combined with greater transparency on research costs and outcomes, would reinvigorate the pharmaceutical market as a driver of both public health and economic growth.

Consumer choice must also be restored to its rightful place as a cornerstone of market-driven healthcare. Patients today lack agency not because they reject capitalism but because the system deprives them of the tools necessary to act as discerning consumers. Reform must focus on expanding access to affordable insurance options, including plans that meet diverse needs and income levels. By reintroducing choice and portability into insurance markets, reforms can empower individuals to select coverage based on value, rather than being tethered to employer-provided plans or navigating limited, costly alternatives. Health savings accounts (HSAs), paired with catastrophic coverage, offer another pathway to expand consumer control while preserving cost-conscious behavior.

Technology and innovation must be leveraged as accelerators of market-driven reform. Digital health tools, telemedicine, and artificial intelligence have already begun to reduce inefficiencies, lower costs, and improve access to care. A competitive market that incentivizes these innovations can amplify their impact, democratizing healthcare delivery while enhancing quality. Policymakers must create an environment that rewards technological advancements without imposing undue regulatory barriers, ensuring that the benefits of innovation reach underserved populations as well as affluent ones. In this context, the market becomes not a source of inequity but a powerful force for expanding access and improving care delivery.

Reforming healthcare through market forces also demands addressing administrative inefficiencies that drain resources and frustrate patients. Streamlining the system through standardized billing processes, interoperable health records, and reduced bureaucratic burdens would eliminate waste while freeing providers to focus on care. When administrative costs are lowered and processes simplified, competition can once again revolve around value and outcomes rather than navigating artificial complexities.

Critics often suggest that market-driven reforms cannot coexist with equity, but this dichotomy is false. A reformed capitalist healthcare system does not have to sacrifice access for the sake of efficiency. By implementing targeted subsidies, tax credits, and safety nets, reforms can ensure that vulnerable populations remain protected while fostering a competitive environment for those who can engage the market fully. Pragmatism lies in designing policies that reconcile market incentives with social responsibility, creating a system that works not only for those who drive economic demand but also for those who rely on its safety nets.

Harnessing market forces for reform demands a strategic recalibration rather than a revolutionary overhaul. The failures of the current system are not inherent to capitalism but stem from its manipulation, misalignment, and fragmentation. By realigning incentives, restoring competition, and empowering consumers, healthcare can be transformed into a system that works for everyone—efficiently, equitably, and sustainably—while maintaining its capitalist foundation. This vision rejects ideological extremes, embracing pragmatic solutions that honor both economic principles and human needs. In doing so, the market becomes not an obstacle to healthcare reform but its most powerful ally.

Expanding Access Through Targeted, Incremental Policies

Expanding access to healthcare requires pragmatic, targeted, and incremental policies that address gaps in affordability and availability without imposing unworkable systemic upheaval. Sweeping, one-size-fits-all reforms often founder under the weight of political opposition and logistical complexity, whereas carefully calibrated measures can steadily widen access while preserving the integrity of the existing framework. A practical path forward acknowledges the limitations of ideology and embraces policy solutions that are feasible, cost-conscious, and rooted in real-world conditions. By focusing on incremental expansion, reforms can create meaningful progress, particularly for underserved populations, without threatening the capitalist foundations of the healthcare system.

Central to this approach is recognizing that access must be improved along multiple fronts: cost, availability, and convenience. The uninsured and underinsured represent the most glaring failure of the current system, but even those with coverage face challenges in accessing care due to geographical disparities, specialist shortages, and prohibitively high out-of-pocket costs. Incremental policies can target these barriers through precision, addressing specific weaknesses without disrupting functioning parts of the system.

One effective strategy is the expansion of subsidies and tax credits for lower- and middle-income individuals, designed to reduce the financial burden of insurance premiums while encouraging greater market participation. Unlike blanket mandates, targeted subsidies respect consumer choice and encourage individuals to select plans suited to their specific needs. Coupled with reforms that reduce deductibles for essential services, this approach would make insurance not only more affordable but also more usable, providing meaningful access to care rather than merely satisfying coverage requirements on paper.

Improving Medicaid's flexibility is another incremental yet impactful measure. While Medicaid already serves as a lifeline for low-income individuals, its rigidity and inconsistent implementation across states create disparities in access and care quality. By incentivizing states to expand eligibility, streamline enrollment processes, and experiment with innovative delivery models, policymakers can broaden Medicaid's reach while maintaining cost efficiency. Programs like premium assistance, which allow Medicaid funds to be used for private insurance, offer an additional pathway to combine public funding with market-based solutions, ensuring that the system remains adaptable and patient-focused.

Expanding access also necessitates addressing provider shortages, particularly in rural and underserved areas where healthcare deserts leave communities without adequate care. Policies that incentivize medical professionals to serve in these regions—such as loan forgiveness programs, financial incentives, and telehealth investments—can close these critical gaps incrementally. Telemedicine, in particular, offers an immediate and scalable solution, allowing patients in isolated areas to connect with providers and specialists without the logistical barriers of travel. By integrating telehealth into mainstream care delivery and expanding reimbursement structures, policymakers can improve access while reducing systemic strain.

Prescription drug access remains another area ripe for targeted reform. High medication costs disproportionately affect vulnerable populations, forcing patients to ration treatment or forgo necessary care. Policies that encourage generic drug production, promote price transparency, and limit anti-competitive practices—such as pay-for-delay agreements—can make medications more affordable without undermining pharmaceutical innovation. Incremental interventions like capping out-of-pocket drug expenses or establishing price-negotiation mechanisms for essential medicines demonstrate that reform does not require abandoning market principles but rather ensuring they work as intended.

For the working uninsured, bridging the gap between employer-based coverage and individual plans is essential. Policies that encourage small businesses to provide insurance—through tax incentives, pooled risk mechanisms, or reinsurance support—can expand employer-based coverage without imposing untenable mandates. Simultaneously, expanding access to health savings accounts (HSAs) provides individuals with additional tools to manage healthcare costs while fostering financial responsibility. Combining HSAs with catastrophic coverage plans creates an affordable safety net that aligns market efficiency with patient needs.

Targeted policies must also recognize that improving access requires addressing inefficiencies that exacerbate cost barriers. Administrative waste, billing complexity, and fragmented care delivery inflate expenses for both providers and patients. Streamlining processes through standardized billing, interoperable electronic health records, and simplified insurance verification systems can reduce overhead costs and redirect resources toward patient care. When combined with reforms that promote preventative care—such as expanding access to screenings, vaccinations, and primary care visits—these measures not only improve access but also generate long-term savings.

Incremental policies succeed where sweeping reforms fail because they work within existing structures rather than seeking to dismantle them. They reflect an understanding of healthcare as an intricate ecosystem that cannot be transformed overnight without unintended consequences. By expanding access through precision and pragmatism, reforms can deliver tangible improvements for those most in need while preserving market-based dynamics that reward innovation, efficiency, and competition. This approach ensures that the healthcare system evolves toward equity and sustainability—not through rhetoric or revolution, but through carefully calibrated progress.

The Role of Technology in Democratizing Healthcare

The role of technology in democratizing healthcare represents one of the most transformative opportunities within a market-based system to improve access, affordability, and quality without necessitating structural upheaval. Technology holds the potential to break down longstanding barriers that have perpetuated disparities, offering tools that allow care to reach underserved populations, streamline processes, and optimize outcomes. When aligned with pragmatic, market-driven reforms, technological innovation becomes a force for both democratization and efficiency, ensuring healthcare is not just available but meaningfully accessible across economic and geographical divides.

The democratizing power of technology lies in its ability to decentralize care delivery, placing the patient at the center of the healthcare ecosystem while diminishing the logistical constraints of location and cost. Telehealth stands as the clearest embodiment of this shift. By enabling virtual consultations, telehealth has fundamentally altered how patients interact with providers, offering convenient, affordable access to care without the burdens of travel or time lost to in-person visits. For rural communities, where provider shortages and healthcare deserts persist, telehealth bridges the gap between need and availability, providing access to specialists and primary care physicians who would otherwise remain out of reach. When supported by targeted reforms, such as expanded reimbursement policies and broadband infrastructure investments, telehealth becomes not a supplement to care but an essential pillar of equitable delivery.

Wearable technologies and mobile health applications further empower patients to take ownership of their healthcare. Devices that monitor vital signs, track chronic conditions, and promote preventive care not only reduce the frequency of emergency interventions but also generate critical data that can improve diagnosis and treatment. From glucose monitors for diabetic patients to heart rate trackers for cardiovascular care, these tools democratize access by shifting the locus of control to individuals, equipping them with real-time insights that enhance engagement and decision-making. When integrated into a broader system of care, these technologies promote early detection and intervention, alleviating downstream costs that burden both patients and providers.

Artificial intelligence (AI) and machine learning represent another transformative frontier, offering solutions to systemic inefficiencies that have long plagued the U.S. healthcare system. AI-powered diagnostics enhance the precision and speed of medical assessments, enabling earlier and more accurate detection of diseases such as cancer, heart conditions, and neurological disorders. By reducing diagnostic errors and optimizing treatment protocols, AI improves both outcomes and cost efficiency. Moreover, machine learning algorithms can analyze vast datasets to identify trends, predict health risks, and streamline resource allocation, ensuring healthcare systems can operate with greater foresight and agility. For patients, these advances translate to improved care delivery that is both responsive and equitable.

Technology also addresses administrative inefficiencies, a persistent source of waste within the U.S. healthcare system. Blockchain solutions for medical records and insurance verification, for example, offer a secure, transparent framework to reduce redundancies and streamline workflows. Electronic health records (EHRs) equipped with AI-powered tools can facilitate care coordination between providers, eliminating fragmented care delivery that leads to unnecessary tests, delays, and costs. When fully optimized, these innovations enhance both the provider and patient experience, freeing resources to be directed toward care rather than bureaucracy.

The affordability of medications and treatments can likewise be improved through technological innovation. Advances in pharmaceutical development—such as AI-driven drug discovery and precision medicine—have the potential to reduce research timelines, lower production costs, and bring life-saving therapies to market more quickly. For patients, particularly those facing chronic illnesses, this means not only broader access to effective treatments but also more personalized therapies that reduce trial-and-error interventions. Technology also fosters transparency in drug pricing, enabling patients to make informed choices and providers to optimize care pathways.

However, the democratization of healthcare through technology requires targeted investment and policy alignment to prevent the exacerbation of existing disparities. Technological solutions cannot succeed if significant portions of the population remain excluded due to economic constraints or infrastructural limitations. Ensuring equitable access to broadband connectivity, expanding insurance coverage for virtual care, and incentivizing the adoption of technology across healthcare systems are critical to realizing its full potential. Similarly, safeguards must be implemented to protect patient privacy and autonomy, ensuring that technological advancement does not come at the expense of ethical principles.

By leveraging technology as a democratizing force, the U.S. healthcare system can achieve a more equitable balance between innovation and accessibility. Pragmatic integration of technological solutions respects the capitalist foundations of the system while addressing its most glaring inefficiencies. Technology does not replace the human element of care; rather, it amplifies its reach, precision, and impact. In doing so, it offers a sustainable pathway to reform—one where patients are empowered, providers are supported, and access to quality care is no longer a privilege but a practical reality.

EQUITY WITHOUT REVOLUTION: BALANCING EFFICIENCY AND FAIRNESS

Equity without revolution requires a delicate reconciliation between fairness and efficiency within the existing capitalist framework of the U.S. healthcare system. The challenge lies in constructing a system that respects market principles while addressing the inequities that leave millions underserved. This balancing act demands pragmatic, incremental reforms that enhance equity without upending the economic engine driving healthcare innovation and delivery. While revolutionary overhauls often appear ideologically appealing, their feasibility and sustainability falter in the face of political resistance, economic disruption, and deeply entrenched institutional interests. Instead, achieving fairness within the current system necessitates targeted strategies that expand access, redistribute resources judiciously, and reorient incentives to align with the public good.

At its core, the pursuit of equity acknowledges the structural barriers that perpetuate disparities in healthcare delivery. Access to care remains stratified along economic, racial, and geographic lines, with marginalized communities disproportionately excluded from preventive services and timely treatment. Incremental reforms can address these divides by optimizing existing structures rather than dismantling them. Programs that expand Medicaid eligibility or provide sliding-scale subsidies for private insurance represent practical steps toward equity, ensuring low-income populations can participate in the healthcare market without sacrificing economic stability. These solutions, grounded in the logic of affordability rather than dependency, build bridges between fairness and fiscal prudence.

Efficiency becomes a vital companion to fairness in a system that must operate within finite resources. Cost containment measures—such as reducing administrative redundancies, negotiating transparent drug pricing, and incentivizing preventive care—create opportunities to reallocate savings toward underserved populations. For instance, preventive health initiatives targeted at chronic conditions like diabetes or hypertension can reduce long-term costs for both individuals and the system at large. By linking efficiency gains to equitable outcomes, reforms can demonstrate that fairness is not antithetical to capitalism but, rather, a necessary evolution for its long-term sustainability.

Insurance market reforms also present opportunities to enhance equity while preserving competition. Policies that incentivize insurers to participate in underserved markets, offer affordable plans, or prioritize coverage for high-risk patients can address gaps without requiring a single-payer overhaul. Innovations like risk pools and reinsurance programs further enable insurers to balance the costs of covering vulnerable populations, ensuring that fairness does not come at the expense of market viability. In this model, equity is achieved through collaboration between public oversight and private innovation, striking a balance that reflects the realities of both economic and social imperatives.

Healthcare equity must also incorporate quality as a measure of fairness. It is insufficient to expand access to care if the care itself remains fragmented, inconsistent, or substandard. Investments in community health centers, telemedicine infrastructure, and rural healthcare initiatives can equalize outcomes across populations, addressing geographic and systemic imbalances. The market, when guided by appropriate incentives, can foster competition that drives improvements in care quality, particularly in regions historically overlooked by large providers. By elevating both access and outcomes, reforms ensure that equity is not reduced to a numbers game but instead reflects tangible improvements in human health.

Technological advancements further provide tools to reconcile fairness and efficiency, democratizing access without demanding structural upheaval. From AI-driven diagnostics that reduce costs to telehealth platforms that bring care to remote areas, technology represents a means of closing gaps that have persisted for decades. By supporting policies that incentivize the adoption of these tools among providers, insurers, and communities, the system can leverage innovation to deliver equitable outcomes. However, safeguards must remain in place to ensure that technological solutions do not reinforce existing divides, particularly for populations with limited access to broadband or digital literacy.

The philosophical underpinning of equity within a capitalist healthcare system rests on a reframing of fairness itself—not as an act of charity but as an economic imperative. Inequities impose systemic costs, whether through emergency care utilization, lost productivity, or the burden of untreated chronic conditions. A fairer healthcare system, therefore, becomes not only a moral obligation but a practical necessity for economic efficiency. By addressing inequities incrementally and pragmatically, reforms safeguard the long-term viability of the healthcare market, ensuring it serves a broader spectrum of the population without collapsing under ideological idealism or financial strain.

Balancing efficiency and fairness requires political will, private sector engagement, and public trust—three pillars that must align to deliver solutions that are both pragmatic and enduring. Revolutionary calls for reform often fracture these alignments, leading to gridlock and stagnation. Incrementalism, by contrast, works within the contours of the system, acknowledging its strengths while remedying its shortcomings. In this balance lies a vision for healthcare that works—not by breaking the system but by evolving it, step by step, toward greater equity and shared prosperity.

A Healthcare Model That Works: The Pragmatic Vision

A healthcare model that works is not one rooted in ideological absolutes or revolutionary upheaval but in pragmatism—a vision that aligns economic incentives, political realities, and social responsibilities. It acknowledges that the United States' healthcare system, for all its flaws, remains a product of unique historical, economic, and cultural forces. Attempting to impose external models wholesale—whether from European single-payer systems or hybrid frameworks elsewhere—overlooks the deep-seated complexities of America's market-driven ethos. Instead, the path forward lies in constructing a model that respects the capitalist foundation while reforming it to deliver better access, efficiency, and equity. This pragmatic vision does not reject the market but reimagines its potential, offering a roadmap for reform that is both functional and sustainable.

At its core, this healthcare model works because it begins with the recognition that access to care is not a zero-sum game. Pragmatic reforms target structural weaknesses without dismantling the economic engine that fuels innovation and choice. Public and private sectors can collaborate rather than conflict, where government policies provide oversight, incentives, and safety nets, while private enterprise drives competition, innovation, and responsiveness to consumer needs. It is not a question of replacing capitalism but of refining it, ensuring that the market serves the interests of patients, not just shareholders.

This vision demands a recalibration of priorities: profit remains a motivating force, but health outcomes and affordability emerge as parallel imperatives.

To achieve this balance, the pragmatic vision embraces incremental yet transformative change. Expanding access through targeted subsidies, risk-sharing mechanisms, and cost containment policies acknowledges that fairness is not achieved overnight but through deliberate, measured reforms. Incrementalism does not mean inaction; it means progress that builds on itself, gaining political and public traction through demonstrable success. A healthcare model that works addresses inefficiencies—administrative waste, opaque pricing, and fragmented care—without resorting to sweeping overhauls that alienate stakeholders or destabilize existing systems. This pragmatism reflects a nuanced understanding of reform's realities: effective change must be adaptable, resilient, and attuned to the varied needs of a diverse population.

Innovation becomes a cornerstone of this vision, with technology positioned as both a disruptor and an equalizer. Tools like AI diagnostics, electronic health records, and telemedicine platforms streamline care delivery, reduce costs, and improve access, particularly for underserved regions. In this model, technology democratizes healthcare while preserving market dynamism, allowing providers to compete not on volume but on value. Public policy accelerates this process through incentives for adoption, ensuring that technological advancements benefit all, not just those who can afford them. Pragmatism acknowledges that the future of healthcare rests in innovation's ability to bridge divides, offering quality care at scale without prohibitive costs.

Efficiency must also be coupled with accountability. A healthcare model that works introduces metrics that measure success not just in economic terms but in health outcomes, patient satisfaction, and equity of access. Transparent pricing, value-based care incentives, and competition-driven improvements hold providers and insurers accountable, shifting the focus from profit extraction to service delivery. Pragmatism ensures that reforms do not punish success or innovation but instead align them with societal benefit. In this vision, profitability becomes synonymous with better health outcomes—a sustainable equilibrium that strengthens the system rather than undermining it.

This model recognizes that true equity is not achieved through universal, one-size-fits-all solutions but through tailored policies that address specific gaps. Rural healthcare, urban underserved populations, and middle-class families facing unaffordable premiums require different interventions. Subsidies, tax incentives, and innovative insurance mechanisms can target these populations with precision, ensuring that incremental changes add up to systemic fairness. By identifying and addressing these gaps pragmatically, the model avoids the ideological rigidity that has stalled reform efforts in the past.

Ultimately, a pragmatic healthcare model succeeds because it respects the political, economic, and cultural forces that shape American life. It does not promise utopia but progress—tangible improvements that restore trust in a system too often viewed as indifferent to human suffering. This vision offers an alternative to both the inertia of rhetoric and the chaos of revolution, positioning healthcare reform as a shared endeavor rather than a battlefield. By aligning market forces with societal priorities, this model achieves what has long seemed impossible: a system that works, not just for those at the top but for everyone it was designed to serve. It is a vision for healthcare that is sustainable, adaptable, and uniquely American—proof that pragmatism, not ideology, is the engine of enduring change.

CHAPTER 14: REIMAGINING RESPONSIBILITY – GOVERNMENT, CORPORATIONS, AND THE INDIVIDUAL

The government serves as both the architect and arbiter of the U.S. healthcare system, a dual role that positions it as the ultimate rule-setter while simultaneously exposing its limitations as an enforcer of accountability. From shaping the foundational structure of healthcare delivery through legislation to providing safety nets for the most vulnerable populations, the government's involvement is expansive but often inconsistent. At its best, it functions as a stabilizing force, crafting policies that expand access to care and regulate markets where corporate interests could otherwise dominate unchecked. At its worst, it becomes an unwieldy actor, paralyzed by political gridlock, influenced by powerful lobbyists, and unable to keep pace with the system's escalating costs and inequities.

The government's regulatory role is evident in the rules it establishes to govern the behavior of private insurers, pharmaceutical companies, and healthcare providers. Through agencies like the Centers for Medicare and Medicaid Services (CMS), the Food and Drug Administration (FDA), and the Centers for Disease Control and Prevention (CDC), it maintains oversight over pricing structures, drug approvals, quality standards, and public health outcomes. While these interventions aim to ensure patient safety and systemic fairness, they frequently fall short in the face of a profit-driven marketplace. For example, Medicare's inability to negotiate drug prices directly with pharmaceutical companies, a consequence of legislative compromises, highlights how policymaking can reinforce corporate power even as it claims to serve the public interest. Regulatory efforts, while well-intentioned, are often fragmented, with state and federal laws creating a patchwork system where accountability and affordability vary dramatically depending on geography.

As a provider, the government fulfills a critical role through public programs like Medicare, Medicaid, and Veterans' Affairs healthcare. These systems serve as lifelines for seniors, low-income families, and military veterans who would otherwise lack access to care. Medicare, introduced in 1965, remains one of the most significant government interventions in U.S. healthcare, offering coverage to tens of millions of older adults and establishing a precedent for state involvement in healthcare funding. Medicaid, in turn, has evolved as a vital, though often underfunded, safety net for low-income individuals, with its impact magnified in states that expanded the program under the Affordable Care Act. Yet, these programs are not without flaws. Inefficiencies, underfunding, and disparities in state implementation create significant gaps in coverage. The Veterans Health Administration, while providing comprehensive care to millions of veterans, has faced repeated scandals involving wait times and systemic mismanagement, illustrating the challenges of delivering care through government bureaucracies.

The political nature of healthcare governance cannot be overlooked. Policymaking in this realm is not merely a matter of pragmatism or public interest; it is a deeply ideological exercise shaped by competing visions of the government's role in society. Conservatives, aligned with free-market principles, often advocate for limited government intervention, favoring deregulation and privatization to foster competition and innovation. Liberals, in contrast, tend to view healthcare as a public good requiring robust government oversight and funding to ensure equitable access. These ideological divides have created a cyclical pattern of reform and rollback, where sweeping changes—such as the Affordable Care Act—are met with fierce resistance, legal challenges, and attempts at dismantlement under subsequent administrations. The result is a system in which long-term stability is elusive, and healthcare remains a political battlefield rather than a policy priority.

The influence of lobbying further complicates the government's ability to act as an impartial arbiter. The healthcare industry—spanning insurers, pharmaceutical companies, hospitals, and provider groups—spends billions annually to shape legislation in its favor. From influencing provisions in major laws to blocking reforms that threaten profits, corporate lobbying often undermines the government's capacity to prioritize public welfare over private gain. The 2003 Medicare Prescription Drug Improvement and Modernization Act, which prohibited Medicare from negotiating drug prices, is a case study in how industry influence can shape policy to the detriment of affordability. Similarly, legislative inertia surrounding surprise medical billing and price transparency reflects the challenges of overcoming industry resistance even in the face of bipartisan public demand.

The government's role in public health adds another dimension to its responsibility. Programs like vaccination campaigns, responses to epidemics, and initiatives promoting preventive care underscore its ability to impact population health outcomes. The COVID-19 pandemic revealed both the strengths and limitations of government intervention, showcasing its capacity to mobilize resources for vaccine development while also exposing gaps in preparedness, coordination, and communication. Public health efforts, though essential, are often underfunded and undervalued, particularly in a system where acute, revenue-generating care is prioritized over prevention.

The government's role as architect and arbiter is marked by contradictions. It wields immense power to shape healthcare's structure and outcomes yet is frequently hindered by political ideologies, lobbying pressures, and bureaucratic inefficiencies. While public programs and regulatory frameworks have expanded access and improved standards of care, they remain incomplete solutions in a system where private interests often outpace public accountability. For the government to fulfill its potential as a stabilizing force, it must reconcile these tensions—asserting its capacity to act as a regulator and provider while resisting the pull of political and corporate inertia. Until then, its efforts will continue to oscillate between progress and stagnation, leaving the healthcare system trapped in a cycle of reform, resistance, and unfinished business.

The Corporate Sector: Balancing Innovation and Profit

The corporate sector occupies a dominant position within the U.S. healthcare system, acting as both a driver of innovation and a primary beneficiary of its profit-driven structure. From pharmaceutical companies to insurance providers, hospital networks to technology firms, corporations form the backbone of a system that is simultaneously admired for its advancements and criticized for its inequities. At its best, the corporate sector fuels cutting-edge medical breakthroughs, expands access to life-saving treatments, and delivers efficient care through economies of scale. At its worst, it prioritizes profits over patients, consolidates power into monopolies, and perpetuates a system where affordability and accessibility remain secondary to shareholder returns.

Pharmaceutical companies stand at the forefront of this dynamic, embodying the dual role of innovator and profiteer. Breakthroughs in drug development have revolutionized the treatment of diseases that were once death sentences—cancer therapies, antiviral medications, and vaccines represent monumental achievements that have extended and improved millions of lives. These advancements, however, come at a cost. Drug pricing in the United States, untethered from global norms, reflects the unchecked influence of pharmaceutical corporations in a system that allows them to maximize profits with limited transparency or accountability. While companies justify high prices as necessary to fund research and development, the reality reveals a more complex picture, where marketing expenditures, shareholder dividends, and executive compensation often eclipse reinvestment in innovation. The hepatitis C drug Sovaldi, for instance, was lauded as a breakthrough treatment but came with a price tag of $1,000 per pill—a cost that left many patients and payers grappling with impossible choices.

In the insurance sector, corporate priorities have shaped how healthcare is accessed and paid for, creating a system in which coverage determines care. Insurers act as intermediaries between patients and providers, managing risk and negotiating costs while ensuring profitability. Private insurance has undoubtedly expanded access to care for many Americans, particularly those with employer-sponsored plans. Yet the system's complexity—marked by deductibles, copayments, and out-of-pocket expenses—has also introduced significant financial burdens. The for-profit model incentivizes insurers to minimize payouts and shift costs onto consumers, resulting in limited coverage, denied claims, and the widespread phenomenon of underinsurance. For those without employer-sponsored plans, the individual insurance market—despite reforms under the Affordable Care Act—remains prohibitively expensive, perpetuating gaps in access for lower-income individuals.

Hospital networks, once community-based institutions, have undergone a transformation fueled by corporate consolidation. Mergers and acquisitions have created sprawling healthcare systems that dominate regional markets, enabling hospitals to wield significant negotiating power with insurers while driving up prices for patients. This consolidation, proponents argue, has led to greater efficiency, improved care coordination, and investments in advanced technologies. Yet it has also fostered monopolistic practices that leave patients and payers with fewer choices and higher costs. Nonprofit hospitals, which make up the majority of facilities, often operate in ways indistinguishable from their for-profit counterparts, prioritizing revenue generation through billing practices that burden patients with exorbitant charges for routine services. Even as hospitals report billions in revenue, many patients emerge from care saddled with unmanageable medical debt—a paradox in which institutions dedicated to healing become agents of financial harm.

Technology companies, too, have entered the healthcare arena, promising to disrupt inefficiencies and transform care delivery. Innovations in artificial intelligence, telemedicine, and health data analytics offer the potential to improve outcomes, reduce costs, and expand access to underserved populations. AI algorithms are streamlining diagnostics, identifying treatment pathways, and personalizing medicine in ways previously unimaginable. Telemedicine has bridged geographical barriers, enabling patients in rural or underserved areas to access care remotely. Yet the integration of technology also raises concerns about equity, as those with limited digital literacy, internet access, or financial means risk being excluded from its benefits. Moreover, the entry of technology giants like Amazon and Google into healthcare raises ethical questions about the commercialization of personal health data and the potential for profit motives to eclipse patient welfare.

While the corporate sector has undeniably driven progress in healthcare, it also bears responsibility for many of the system's structural failures. The relentless pursuit of profit has led to practices that prioritize financial outcomes over patient care—surprise medical billing, opaque pricing structures, and the overutilization of high-margin services reflect a system designed to extract value from patients rather than deliver it. The influence of corporate lobbying further exacerbates these issues, ensuring that policies align with industry interests rather than public needs. Attempts to regulate drug prices, enforce price transparency, or curtail monopolistic practices have faced formidable opposition from industry stakeholders determined to protect their profit margins.

The tension between innovation and profit lies at the heart of the corporate sector's role in healthcare. While companies have produced groundbreaking advancements that save lives and push the boundaries of medicine, their prioritization of revenue over equity has left millions of Americans without affordable access to care. The challenge moving forward is not to dismantle the corporate presence within healthcare but to reimagine its role—aligning innovation with accountability, profits with patient outcomes. This requires a system in which corporations are incentivized not merely to maximize shareholder returns but to deliver value in ways that balance financial sustainability with the broader imperative of equitable care. Until this balance is achieved, the corporate sector will remain both the engine of healthcare's greatest successes and the source of its most glaring failures.

THE INDIVIDUAL: ACCOUNTABILITY IN HEALTH AND WELLNESS

The individual's role in the U.S. healthcare system is deeply intertwined with the nation's foundational ethos of personal responsibility and self-determination. The expectation that individuals should take ownership of their health—making choices that promote wellness, prevent illness, and navigate the healthcare system effectively—reflects a broader cultural emphasis on autonomy and accountability. However, this ideal of personal responsibility often masks the complex realities that shape individual health outcomes, including socioeconomic barriers, systemic inequities, and the overwhelming influence of external forces such as corporate practices, environmental factors, and public policy decisions.

At its core, the emphasis on individual accountability suggests that health is largely a matter of lifestyle choices. Eat well, exercise regularly, avoid smoking and excessive alcohol consumption, and the likelihood of developing chronic diseases diminishes. Public health campaigns have reinforced this message for decades, encouraging preventive behaviors as a means of reducing personal and societal burdens. The growing wellness industry, with its proliferation of fitness programs, nutritional supplements, wearable health trackers, and self-care regimens, has further entrenched the narrative that individuals have control over their health outcomes. For many, these tools represent empowerment, allowing individuals to take a proactive approach to their well-being. Yet this framework, while valid to a degree, oversimplifies the relationship between individual behavior and health outcomes, failing to account for the significant disparities in access to resources that enable such choices.

The reality is far more complex. Health cannot be reduced to a series of personal decisions when those decisions are constrained by social and economic circumstances. Individuals from marginalized or lower-income communities often lack access to nutritious food, safe neighborhoods for exercise, quality healthcare services, and the financial stability needed to prioritize wellness. The prevalence of food deserts in urban and rural areas, where fresh produce and healthy options are unavailable, forces many families to rely on inexpensive, processed foods. Employment insecurity and stagnant wages may leave individuals with neither the time nor the means to engage in preventive care or wellness activities. These disparities reveal the limits of personal responsibility as a guiding principle, highlighting the need for structural changes that address the systemic barriers preventing individuals from making healthier choices.

Furthermore, the notion of individual accountability can quickly shift into blame when illness occurs. Chronic diseases like diabetes, heart disease, and obesity are often framed as the result of poor personal choices rather than the outcome of complex interactions between genetics, environment, and systemic inequalities. This perception fosters stigma, eroding empathy for those who suffer and shifting attention away from the broader systems that contribute to poor health. The privatized nature of the U.S. healthcare system exacerbates this dynamic, as individuals bear financial responsibility for their care through copays, deductibles, and out-of-pocket expenses. Those unable to afford necessary treatments are often left to navigate illness alone, their suffering framed as a consequence of personal failings rather than a systemic failure of access and affordability.

Compounding this challenge is the difficulty of navigating a healthcare system designed for those with the time, resources, and knowledge to advocate for themselves. The complexities of insurance policies, billing practices, and provider networks require individuals to act as their own healthcare advocates—a role for which many are unprepared. For those with lower health literacy or limited English proficiency, the system's opacity can become insurmountable, leaving them without care or drowning in medical debt. In this environment, personal accountability becomes a burden disproportionately placed on those least equipped to shoulder it.

Yet personal responsibility, when properly supported, remains an essential component of any healthcare system. Preventive care, lifestyle changes, and informed decision-making can significantly reduce the burden of chronic disease, improve quality of life, and lower healthcare costs for individuals and society. Achieving this, however, requires more than admonishing individuals to "do better." It demands policies and cultural shifts that empower individuals to take control of their health by ensuring they have the resources, education, and support to do so. Employers can play a role through workplace wellness programs, flexible schedules for preventive care, and mental health support. Governments can invest in public health infrastructure, education campaigns, and community-based interventions that make healthy living more accessible. Healthcare providers must move beyond treating illness to fostering long-term relationships with patients that prioritize preventive care and shared decision-making.

Equally important is the need to address the cultural attitudes that underpin personal responsibility. A shift is required toward viewing health as a shared societal responsibility rather than an individual burden. This means fostering an environment in which individuals are encouraged to make healthy choices not out of fear of blame or financial ruin but because they are supported by systems that make those choices viable and sustainable. Education plays a crucial role here, as health literacy remains a key determinant of an individual's ability to navigate the system, understand risks, and engage in preventive care. Schools, workplaces, and community organizations must prioritize health education that empowers individuals to take proactive steps toward wellness.

The role of the individual in healthcare is both undeniable and deeply contextual. Personal accountability must be reimagined not as an isolated demand but as a shared commitment between individuals, corporations, and governments. The individual cannot succeed in achieving wellness if the systems around them are designed to fail. Addressing this requires a recalibration of priorities: a recognition that while individuals bear responsibility for their choices, society bears responsibility for ensuring that those choices are meaningful and attainable. Only through this shared responsibility can the nation begin to bridge the gap between health as a privilege for the few and health as a right for all.

Toward Shared Responsibility: Bridging Stakeholder Roles

The future of healthcare in America hinges on a fundamental shift toward shared responsibility—a recalibration of how government, corporations, and individuals align their roles to create a more equitable, sustainable, and functional system. While each stakeholder has a distinct role to play, the entrenched fragmentation between them has perpetuated a system in which accountability is displaced, incentives are misaligned, and those who are most vulnerable are left behind. Bridging these roles demands both structural reforms and a cultural transformation—an acknowledgment that healthcare is not just an individual or market-driven concern but a shared societal obligation.

The government, as both architect and arbiter, must reclaim its place as a steward of public health. While market forces have driven innovation, they have also amplified inequities, requiring the state to step in as a counterbalance. This does not necessitate a complete overhaul of the existing capitalist infrastructure but rather a strategic intervention to close gaps, protect vulnerable populations, and realign incentives. Governments at all levels must prioritize health as a public good by investing in accessible infrastructure, expanding preventive care initiatives, and regulating corporate practices that exploit the most basic human need. Policy frameworks that reward innovation while holding corporations accountable for affordability and equity can create a system where profit and care are no longer at odds. However, such changes will require a departure from the political gridlock that has long stymied progress, necessitating bipartisan recognition that healthcare inefficiencies harm not only individuals but the broader economic and social fabric of the nation.

Corporate stakeholders—pharmaceutical companies, insurers, providers, and technology firms—must also embrace a more balanced approach to their dual role as innovators and profiteers. While the pursuit of profit is intrinsic to their existence, it is no longer sufficient to measure success solely by quarterly earnings. Instead, corporations must recognize their ethical and economic stake in fostering long-term health outcomes. When chronic disease proliferates unchecked, or entire demographics are priced out of care, the resulting burden on the system undermines its stability and sustainability. Companies that invest in value-based care models—where incentives are tied to health outcomes rather than volume of services—demonstrate that profitability and patient well-being can coexist. Similarly, insurers and employers can lead efforts to address the social determinants of health, funding programs that reduce barriers to care and promote wellness among their customers and employees. These shifts will not occur without significant pressure from both policymakers and consumers, but they represent a critical step in bridging the chasm between corporate profit motives and societal well-being.

The individual, too, must play a pivotal role, but in a manner that acknowledges the complexity of personal accountability. For too long, the narrative of individual responsibility has been wielded as both a virtue and a weapon, placing undue blame on those who fall ill while ignoring the systemic barriers they face. Reimagining personal accountability requires a paradigm shift: individuals must be empowered, not shamed, to prioritize their health. This means creating environments in which healthy choices are accessible, affordable, and sustainable. Preventive care, nutritional education, mental health support, and health literacy programs are essential tools in enabling individuals to take control of their well-being. However, personal responsibility cannot exist in isolation. For individuals to succeed in managing their health, they must be supported by policies that guarantee access to care, workplaces that prioritize wellness, and communities that foster healthier lifestyles.

The true challenge—and opportunity—lies in fostering synergy between these stakeholders. A shared responsibility model requires government intervention that empowers individuals without stifling corporate innovation, corporate practices that prioritize long-term health outcomes without sacrificing financial sustainability, and individual engagement that thrives under systemic support.

Such alignment is not utopian; it has been demonstrated in localized efforts across the country, where public-private partnerships have improved access, reduced costs, and delivered better outcomes. For example, community health initiatives funded by corporate stakeholders and supported by state and federal policies have successfully reduced rates of preventable diseases in underserved populations. Similarly, models like accountable care organizations (ACOs) provide a blueprint for aligning incentives between providers, insurers, and patients to prioritize value over volume.

At its heart, the shift toward shared responsibility represents a cultural reckoning with the values that underpin the healthcare system. The U.S. must confront the contradictions inherent in a model that celebrates individualism while relying on collective resources to sustain its infrastructure. This requires a redefinition of success—not just for governments and corporations but for society as a whole. Success must be measured not by the profitability of healthcare industries alone but by the health outcomes of the population they serve. It must recognize that a system designed to prioritize care, innovation, and equity is not a threat to capitalism but a necessary evolution of it.

Bridging stakeholder roles in healthcare is about creating a system in which responsibility is not avoided or displaced but shared and aligned for the common good. Governments must lead with policies that protect and empower; corporations must innovate with an eye toward equitable access; and individuals must be supported in their pursuit of better health. Only through this collective effort can the U.S. healthcare system move beyond its current paradox—transforming from a fragmented, profit-driven enterprise into a model of shared accountability that balances care, innovation, and sustainability.

Chapter 15: The Cost of Inaction

The price of stagnation in the U.S. healthcare system is not a hypothetical question but a reality unfolding in real time. Each day that the system remains untouched by meaningful reform, the weight of its inefficiencies and inequities grows heavier, pressing down on individuals, families, businesses, and the broader economy. What might seem like an absence of action is, in truth, a deliberate decision to maintain a fractured system that serves some at the expense of many. The costs—economic, social, and moral—are mounting, with ripple effects that extend far beyond the domain of healthcare, infiltrating the foundations of American society.

Economically, the status quo is a slow bleed, draining resources from every corner of the country. Households feel this strain most acutely, with millions struggling to pay for life-saving medications or delaying essential treatments due to cost. The rise of medical debt is staggering, with countless families one unexpected illness away from financial ruin. Employers, too, bear the burden, forced to shoulder skyrocketing insurance premiums that leave less room for innovation, growth, or fair employee compensation. On a national scale, the unsustainable trajectory of healthcare spending—already outpacing inflation and GDP growth—threatens the very solvency of public programs like Medicare and Medicaid.

Yet the economic burden tells only part of the story. Socially, the impact of inaction is eroding the fabric of communities, creating sharp divides between those with access to high-quality care and those left behind. Healthcare inequities—especially stark along lines of race, income, and geography—are not merely statistics but daily realities for millions of Americans. For some, the nearest hospital may be hours away; for others, an overburdened emergency room serves as their primary source of care. These disparities deepen cycles of poverty and illness, reinforcing a grim reality where a person's health is too often determined by their zip code.

The moral dimension of this crisis cannot be overstated. A system that allows preventable suffering and death, while enriching a select few, calls into question the values upon which it is built. Public trust, already fragile, is further undermined by stories of patients denied necessary treatments or burdened with ruinous bills after surviving catastrophic illnesses. The enduring failures of the system are not abstract flaws; they are lived experiences that erode faith in institutions, leaving people disillusioned and angry.

Even as these costs pile up, the opportunity for meaningful change grows more elusive. The longer systemic reform is delayed, the harder it becomes to untangle the web of entrenched interests that profit from the current structure. Lobbyists for pharmaceutical companies, private insurers, and hospital conglomerates ensure that legislative gridlock persists, protecting their margins while ordinary Americans continue to pay the price. This inertia has consequences far beyond healthcare, fostering a culture of cynicism and complacency that permeates the political landscape.

To maintain the status quo is to choose a path of least resistance, but it is not without consequence. The price is paid in dollars and lives, in the untapped potential of people who might have thrived if only they had access to the care they needed. It is a cost borne by the nation as a whole, its reputation as a leader in innovation and opportunity tarnished by a system that prioritizes profit over people. As the cracks widen, the question becomes not whether the system will break under its weight, but when—and who will suffer most when it does.

ECONOMIC BURDEN OF THE STATUS QUO

The economic burden of maintaining the status quo in the U.S. healthcare system is a paradox of staggering costs and diminishing returns. As healthcare spending balloons to nearly 20% of GDP, it becomes increasingly clear that the financial strain is unsustainable, yet the outcomes fail to reflect the exorbitant price tag. The economic toll reverberates through households, businesses, and government budgets, exposing a system where inefficiency and inequity compound to create a fiscal crisis disguised as routine.

For individuals and families, the economic weight of the current system is both immediate and long-term. Out-of-pocket expenses for premiums, copays, and medications continue to rise, pushing many Americans into medical debt that can take years, even decades, to repay. The numbers are stark: millions of families are forced to choose between basic necessities and critical healthcare. In this landscape, even insured individuals are not immune to financial catastrophe, with surprise billing and denied claims adding layers of uncertainty to an already precarious situation. These pressures do not merely cause financial strain; they diminish quality of life, stifle upward mobility, and perpetuate cycles of poverty.

The ripple effect extends to businesses, which bear the brunt of rising insurance costs for their employees. Employer-sponsored health insurance, long a cornerstone of American coverage, has become a double-edged sword. Companies must navigate ever-increasing premiums, which erode profits and leave less room for competitive wages, research and development, and expansion. Small businesses are particularly vulnerable, often unable to afford comprehensive coverage, leaving their employees with limited options. The result is a workforce that is financially overburdened and, in many cases, less productive due to untreated health conditions.

At the governmental level, the financial implications are equally dire. Public programs like Medicare and Medicaid consume an ever-growing portion of state and federal budgets, with spending projections showing no signs of abating. As these programs strain under the weight of an aging population and rising healthcare costs, the pressure to fund them crowds out other critical investments in infrastructure, education, and social services. The inefficiencies within the system exacerbate the problem, with administrative waste, inflated prices, and opaque billing practices consuming billions that could be redirected toward care.

The macroeconomic consequences of these dynamics are profound. The United States spends more on healthcare per capita than any other nation, yet its health outcomes—such as life expectancy and chronic disease management—lag behind those of its peers. This disparity represents a profound misallocation of resources, where vast sums are funneled into profits for insurers, pharmaceutical companies, and hospital conglomerates rather than improving patient care. The opportunity costs are staggering; the money spent propping up this system could be used to address pressing societal challenges, from combating climate change to advancing technological innovation.

Inaction perpetuates a vicious cycle. As costs rise, access becomes more restricted, leading to delayed or foregone care that ultimately results in higher expenses down the line. Chronic illnesses that could have been managed or prevented in their early stages escalate into emergencies, requiring expensive interventions that strain both individuals and the system. The lack of preventive care, driven by cost barriers, only adds to the long-term economic burden, ensuring that the status quo is not just expensive but self-perpetuating.

The economic burden of inaction is not just a ledger of rising costs; it is a reflection of misplaced priorities and squandered potential. Each dollar spent maintaining this broken system represents a lost opportunity to build a healthier, more equitable, and more sustainable future. If the financial trajectory remains unchecked, it will not only undermine economic stability but also compromise the very ideals of fairness and opportunity that the American healthcare system purports to serve.

SOCIAL INEQUITIES AND PUBLIC HEALTH DECLINE

The social inequities embedded within the U.S. healthcare system are both a symptom and a cause of broader societal disparities, creating a feedback loop that perpetuates cycles of disadvantage. When access to healthcare is dictated by socioeconomic status, racial identity, or geographic location, the consequences reverberate far beyond the individual, affecting families, communities, and the nation as a whole. The cost of maintaining the status quo in this regard is immeasurable, manifesting in public health crises, reduced social cohesion, and a profound erosion of trust in the system.

At its core, the current healthcare model exacerbates existing inequalities. Low-income populations, disproportionately represented by marginalized racial and ethnic groups, often find themselves in healthcare deserts—areas with limited access to quality medical facilities or providers. These communities face higher rates of preventable diseases, lower life expectancy, and limited access to preventive care. The inequities are stark: an individual's zip code can be as predictive of their health outcomes as their genetic code. The lack of accessible healthcare reinforces economic and social barriers, trapping individuals in cycles of poor health and financial instability.

Public health, which thrives on equitable access to care, suffers dramatically under these conditions. Preventable illnesses, such as diabetes, hypertension, and certain cancers, are allowed to flourish unchecked in vulnerable populations, creating a public health burden that spills over into the broader community. Outbreaks of communicable diseases, for example, disproportionately affect underserved areas but do not remain confined there. The lack of a cohesive public health strategy, rooted in equitable access, leaves the entire population vulnerable to systemic risks.

The ramifications of inaction extend to mental health, an often-overlooked dimension of public health. Marginalized communities frequently face higher rates of trauma, stress, and mental illness, yet they are among the least likely to receive appropriate care. Stigmatization, coupled with inadequate funding for mental health services, ensures that the emotional and psychological toll of inequality remains unaddressed. This neglect not only diminishes individual well-being but also leads to societal costs, including increased homelessness, incarceration, and substance abuse.

The decline in public health is further aggravated by the economic pressures discussed earlier, as delayed or forgone care due to financial constraints leads to more severe health conditions. The inability to afford routine check-ups or medications pushes individuals to rely on emergency care as a last resort. This reactive approach to healthcare places immense strain on hospitals and emergency services, driving up costs and diverting resources away from preventive measures. The cycle is both inefficient and deeply inequitable, with the most vulnerable populations bearing the brunt of its failures.

On a societal level, these inequities undermine trust in institutions. When entire segments of the population feel excluded from the promise of quality healthcare, it fosters resentment and alienation. This erosion of trust has broader implications for democracy and social stability, as people become disillusioned with a system they perceive as rigged against them. Healthcare inequities, therefore, are not just a medical or economic issue; they are a moral and political one, reflecting the priorities and values of the society that sustains them.

The public health decline fueled by these inequities affects everyone, not just those directly marginalized by the system. The rise in chronic diseases, preventable illnesses, and mental health crises creates a national burden that drains resources and limits collective potential. Addressing these issues requires a shift in focus from profit-driven models to community-oriented solutions. Without action, the societal costs will continue to escalate, leaving behind not just individuals but the very fabric of the nation's health and well-being.

IMPACT ON HEALTHCARE PROVIDERS AND WORKFORCE

The ramifications of a stagnant and inequitable healthcare system extend deeply into the lives of healthcare providers and the workforce that sustains it. While patients bear the brunt of systemic shortcomings, the individuals tasked with delivering care are increasingly overburdened, under-resourced, and demoralized. The status quo perpetuates a cycle in which healthcare workers are forced to navigate a system that prioritizes financial metrics over patient outcomes, leading to burnout, workforce attrition, and declining morale. This growing crisis within the healthcare workforce not only affects providers themselves but also compromises the quality and accessibility of care across the nation.

One of the most pressing issues is the pervasive burnout among healthcare providers. Physicians, nurses, and other medical professionals face relentless demands in a system structured around productivity quotas, administrative burdens, and insufficient staffing levels. The emphasis on meeting insurance-driven metrics—such as patient throughput and billing targets—diverts attention from patient-centered care, eroding the professional satisfaction that drew many to the field in the first place. Studies consistently show alarmingly high rates of burnout, depression, and even suicide among healthcare workers, a stark indicator of the system's toll on its most essential contributors.

The administrative complexity of the U.S. healthcare system compounds this burden. Providers often spend hours navigating insurance approvals, coding requirements, and billing disputes, detracting from the time they can dedicate to direct patient care. For many, the frustration of being bogged down in paperwork rather than practicing medicine fosters a sense of disillusionment.

This bureaucratic overload is particularly acute in underserved areas, where providers must stretch limited resources to cover an overwhelming volume of patients with complex needs, often without adequate support.

The impact of these challenges is not limited to the individual provider; it ripples throughout the entire healthcare workforce. High turnover rates among nurses, physicians, and support staff disrupt continuity of care and strain already limited resources. Hospitals and clinics face mounting costs associated with recruiting and training replacements, while remaining staff are left to shoulder even greater workloads. The loss of experienced professionals diminishes institutional knowledge and undermines the capacity to deliver high-quality care, especially in rural and low-income areas where shortages are most acute.

These workforce pressures also exacerbate disparities in access to care. Burnout and dissatisfaction are particularly pronounced among providers serving marginalized communities, where the challenges of addressing complex social determinants of health are compounded by resource limitations. As a result, these areas are often the first to experience provider shortages, further entrenching healthcare inequities. The cycle becomes self-perpetuating: inadequate support leads to workforce attrition, which in turn diminishes access to care, worsening patient outcomes and increasing provider stress.

The systemic neglect of healthcare workers has broader implications for public health and national resilience. In times of crisis—such as pandemics or natural disasters—the fragility of the workforce becomes glaringly apparent. The COVID-19 pandemic, for example, exposed the vulnerabilities of an overstretched system, with providers facing unprecedented challenges while grappling with inadequate protections, insufficient supplies, and unsustainable workloads. The lessons of such crises remain unheeded if the structural deficiencies that burden the workforce are not addressed.

Maintaining the status quo risks driving the healthcare system toward a breaking point, where workforce shortages, burnout, and declining morale render it incapable of meeting even basic needs. Addressing these challenges requires systemic reform that prioritizes the well-being of providers alongside patients. This includes reducing administrative burdens, ensuring equitable distribution of resources, and fostering a culture that values care over profit. Without such changes, the healthcare workforce will continue to bear the weight of an untenable system, to the detriment of providers and patients alike.

EROSION OF TRUST IN INSTITUTIONS

The persistence of systemic failures in healthcare not only deepens economic and social divides but also erodes public trust in the institutions that shape and sustain the system. Trust, a foundational element of any functioning society, is critical in healthcare, where vulnerable individuals rely on professionals, insurers, and policymakers to prioritize their well-being. Yet, as inequities widen, costs spiral, and inefficiencies persist, the credibility of these institutions diminishes, leaving patients and communities skeptical of their intentions and capabilities. The erosion of trust reverberates beyond the healthcare system, undermining societal cohesion and democratic governance.

Patients, particularly those from marginalized or economically disadvantaged backgrounds, are often the first to lose faith in healthcare institutions. For those repeatedly denied access to care due to cost or insurance barriers, the system ceases to be a source of support and becomes an adversary. Stories of life-saving treatments denied due to pre-existing conditions or financial constraints amplify perceptions of a system designed to protect corporate profits over individual lives. These experiences foster cynicism, resentment, and a sense of helplessness that erodes the foundational trust between patients and providers.

The opacity of pricing and billing practices further aggravates this distrust. Patients frequently encounter unexpected medical bills, inflated charges, and bewildering cost structures that leave them feeling deceived and exploited. For many, the lack of transparency symbolizes a deeper disregard for fairness and accountability, as institutions prioritize financial gain over equitable care. This mistrust extends to insurers and pharmaceutical companies, whose roles in perpetuating high costs and limiting coverage are increasingly scrutinized by the public.

Healthcare providers, too, grapple with declining trust—not only in the systems they work within but also in the patients they serve. Providers report frustration with administrative processes, insurance constraints, and the pressure to prioritize productivity over personalized care. This disconnect undermines the patient-provider relationship, as both parties navigate a system that often pits their interests against one another. The result is a breakdown in communication, collaboration, and mutual understanding—essential elements of effective healthcare delivery.

The erosion of trust in healthcare institutions also spills over into public confidence in government and policy-making. Legislative failures to address systemic inequities or rein in corporate power fuel perceptions of a political system captured by special interests. This disillusionment is compounded by highly partisan debates on healthcare reform, which often prioritize ideological victories over substantive solutions. When the public sees little progress in addressing healthcare's persistent challenges, skepticism about the government's ability—or willingness—to act grows, contributing to broader disengagement from democratic processes.

A decline in trust also hampers the implementation of public health initiatives. Vaccine hesitancy, for instance, is often rooted in mistrust of pharmaceutical companies, government agencies, and healthcare providers. In a landscape where institutions are viewed with suspicion, even well-intentioned efforts to promote health and safety are met with resistance, jeopardizing collective well-being. The COVID-19 pandemic offered a stark illustration of how fractured trust can undermine public health responses, with misinformation and institutional skepticism hindering vaccination campaigns and compliance with preventive measures.

Rebuilding trust requires systemic change that goes beyond superficial gestures. It demands transparency in pricing and decision-making, accountability for inequities, and a commitment to prioritizing patient outcomes over profits. Empowering communities through accessible, equitable care and fostering meaningful engagement between providers and patients are critical steps in restoring confidence. Without these measures, the erosion of trust will continue to deepen, leaving individuals and communities increasingly disconnected from the institutions meant to serve them. The stakes extend far beyond healthcare, as the loss of trust in such a vital sector weakens the fabric of society itself, perpetuating cycles of alienation and disempowerment.

GLOBAL REPERCUSSIONS AND MISSED OPPORTUNITIES

The consequences of inaction in the U.S. healthcare system ripple far beyond national borders, carrying global implications and representing missed opportunities for leadership, innovation, and collaboration. As one of the world's largest economies and a prominent player in shaping international health policy, the United States' approach to healthcare is scrutinized, emulated, and critiqued worldwide. Yet, the persistence of inefficiencies, inequities, and exorbitant costs undermines its credibility as a global leader in advancing health systems and addressing cross-border challenges. By failing to address its domestic shortcomings, the U.S. forfeits the chance to set a positive example and leverage its influence for global progress.

One key repercussion is the missed opportunity to contribute meaningfully to global health equity. Despite significant advancements in medical technology and pharmaceutical innovation, the U.S. healthcare system often prioritizes profit over accessibility, creating barriers that extend to international partnerships. For instance, the high costs of U.S.-developed treatments and medications make them inaccessible not only to many Americans but also to countries in the Global South. This disparity exacerbates global health inequalities, as nations with fewer resources struggle to access critical innovations that could improve or save lives. The perception of the U.S. as a health innovator is thus overshadowed by its role in perpetuating a model that prioritizes markets over humanity.

Furthermore, the systemic inefficiencies of the U.S. healthcare system diminish its capacity to engage in global health crises effectively. When domestic infrastructure is overwhelmed by rising costs, understaffing, and inequitable access, the country is less equipped to mobilize resources for global emergencies such as pandemics, natural disasters, or refugee health crises. The COVID-19 pandemic revealed how internal disarray undermines international cooperation, with the U.S. struggling to balance its domestic response with global obligations. This lack of preparedness not only weakens America's leadership but also impedes collective efforts to address transnational threats to health and security.

The U.S. also risks falling behind in the global race for healthcare innovation. Countries with more equitable and efficient systems, such as those in Scandinavia or East Asia, have demonstrated how universal access and investment in public health yield better outcomes and foster economic stability. By clinging to a profit-driven model, the U.S. limits its potential to harness the full power of its research institutions, private enterprises, and public health agencies. Collaborative opportunities with countries that prioritize universal access are often underexplored, as ideological divides and systemic inefficiencies hinder the ability to integrate best practices or co-develop transformative solutions.

Another missed opportunity lies in global influence. The U.S. has long wielded soft power through its cultural, economic, and technological leadership, but the healthcare system's glaring shortcomings undermine this advantage. In international diplomacy, credibility matters, and the inability to provide affordable, equitable care to its population weakens the U.S.'s position in advocating for human rights, including the right to health. Nations that look to the U.S. for guidance may instead turn to countries with more inclusive healthcare models, diminishing America's role as a benchmark for development and governance.

Global health partnerships, too, are affected by the U.S.'s internal healthcare struggles. Multinational initiatives aimed at combating infectious diseases, improving maternal and child health, or expanding access to vaccines often require both financial and logistical leadership. When the U.S. channels substantial resources into a fragmented, inefficient domestic system, its ability to contribute to these initiatives is constrained. This dynamic not only limits global progress but also hinders the U.S. from capitalizing on the goodwill and strategic alliances that such contributions foster.

Addressing the systemic flaws in the U.S. healthcare system is not merely a domestic imperative—it is a global responsibility. A more equitable, efficient, and accessible healthcare model would enhance the U.S.'s capacity to lead in international health initiatives, share innovations that benefit humanity, and respond decisively to global crises. By tackling the barriers that hinder reform, the U.S. has the potential to redefine its role on the world stage, transforming from a cautionary tale of inequality to a beacon of possibility. The stakes of inaction are not confined to American borders; they are felt in missed chances to shape a healthier, more interconnected world.

The Peril of Indifference

Indifference to the shortcomings of the healthcare system poses one of the gravest risks to a nation's well-being, both socially and economically. When systemic flaws are met with apathy or resignation, the consequences extend beyond immediate challenges to erode the foundational principles of equity, trust, and progress. The peril of indifference lies in its quiet, insidious nature: it normalizes dysfunction, stifles reform, and allows the burden of an inadequate system to grow unchecked. In the case of U.S. healthcare, such indifference not only perpetuates suffering but also cements barriers to achieving a more just and effective system.

At the heart of this indifference is a societal desensitization to the inequities and inefficiencies that plague the system. When stories of medical bankruptcies, unaffordable prescriptions, and delayed treatments become commonplace, they risk losing their capacity to shock or inspire action. This normalization breeds complacency, fostering a collective tolerance for what should be intolerable. Indifference acts as a societal anesthetic, dulling the urgency to address disparities and allowing inertia to take precedence over progress. Over time, it reinforces the perception that meaningful change is either unattainable or unnecessary.

For policymakers, indifference manifests as political paralysis. Without sustained public pressure or widespread outrage, the incentive to pursue bold reforms diminishes. The complex and contentious nature of healthcare policy requires both political will and public engagement, but indifference undermines both. Lawmakers may view healthcare reform as a politically risky endeavor, especially in a polarized environment where entrenched interests resist change. As a result, incremental fixes become the norm, addressing symptoms rather than root causes and leaving the system increasingly fragmented and unsustainable.

The economic costs of indifference are equally profound. A healthcare system left to stagnate under the weight of inefficiencies drains resources that could otherwise fuel innovation, education, and infrastructure. Employers face rising insurance costs that stifle competitiveness, workers struggle with medical debt that limits spending power, and communities bear the financial strain of untreated illnesses that escalate into public health crises. Indifference to these economic realities perpetuates a cycle of waste and underperformance, undermining the nation's long-term prosperity.

Socially, indifference deepens divisions and fosters inequality. In a system where access to care is often determined by income, geography, or employment status, the failure to act exacerbates disparities that undermine social cohesion. Communities already marginalized by systemic inequities bear a disproportionate share of the burden, leading to poorer health outcomes, shorter life expectancies, and diminished opportunities for upward mobility. Indifference to these realities not only perpetuates injustice but also erodes the social fabric that binds communities together.

Perhaps the most troubling consequence of indifference is its impact on hope and agency. When individuals feel powerless to influence change, apathy takes root, creating a vicious cycle of disengagement. The belief that the system is impervious to reform discourages advocacy and innovation, further entrenching the status quo. This resignation undermines democratic principles, as citizens withdraw from the processes and institutions meant to serve them. In this environment, even well-intentioned efforts to advance healthcare reform face uphill battles, hindered by a lack of public momentum and support.

The peril of indifference extends to future generations, who inherit a system weakened by neglect. The longer systemic flaws go unaddressed, the harder they become to resolve. Rising costs, aging populations, and evolving health challenges compound the urgency for action, yet indifference delays the investments and reforms necessary to prepare for these inevitabilities. Without intervention, the next generation will face an even more fragmented, inequitable, and unsustainable system—a legacy of neglect that could have been avoided.

Confronting the peril of indifference requires a collective awakening to the moral, social, and economic imperatives for reform. It demands that society refuse to accept suffering and inequity as inevitable, and that individuals recognize their power to advocate for change. In the face of indifference, the most profound act of resistance is engagement—an active commitment to envisioning and building a healthcare system that reflects the values of justice, dignity, and compassion. Without this commitment, the status quo becomes a self-fulfilling prophecy, ensuring that the cost of inaction continues to rise.

A Healthcare System America Deserves

The U.S. healthcare system, with all its intricacies and contradictions, stands as a powerful reflection of the nation itself. It embodies the hallmarks of American identity: a relentless drive for innovation, a deep-rooted belief in individualism, and an unapologetic embrace of capitalism. At its best, it is a world leader in pioneering medical advancements, delivering groundbreaking treatments and fostering an ecosystem where cutting-edge technologies flourish. Yet, these achievements coexist with glaring inequities, inefficiencies, and systemic failures, creating a paradox that is uniquely American.

This system, far from being a chaotic accident, operates as it was designed—a finely tuned machine for prioritizing profit, competition, and market-driven solutions. It rewards the enterprising and the resourceful, offering extraordinary care for those who can afford it while leaving others to navigate an often inaccessible and bewildering landscape. Much like the broader economy, the healthcare system thrives on innovation but often struggles to distribute its benefits equitably.

Healthcare in the United States is not merely a service or an industry; it is a lens through which the nation's values and priorities are magnified. Its successes and failures are not isolated but deeply interwoven with the ideologies that define American life. The triumphs of specialized medicine and entrepreneurial breakthroughs speak to the country's capacity for ingenuity and resilience. However, the persistent disparities in access and outcomes highlight a darker truth: the system's reliance on market dynamics has systematically marginalized those who cannot compete within its framework.

In this way, the healthcare system functions as a microcosm of America itself—dynamic and innovative yet stratified and unequal. It challenges the nation to reconcile its proudest ideals with its starkest realities, asking whether it can chart a future that honors its spirit of ingenuity without sacrificing its commitment to fairness and shared progress.

REFRAMING THE NARRATIVE AROUND HEALTHCARE

To truly understand and address the challenges of the U.S. healthcare system, the prevailing narrative must be reframed. For too long, discussions have centered on the binary of a "broken" system versus an unattainable ideal. This perspective oversimplifies the reality: the system is not malfunctioning but functioning precisely as it was designed—prioritizing innovation and profit within the framework of a market-driven economy. The question is not whether the system works but for whom it works and at what cost.

By shifting the conversation from dysfunction to design, we can uncover opportunities for meaningful reform. Acknowledging the system's successes—its unmatched ability to drive medical breakthroughs and deliver exceptional care in specific contexts—allows for a more balanced critique. These strengths are not incidental; they are direct outcomes of the competitive forces embedded in the healthcare framework. Yet, these same forces often exacerbate inequities, leaving millions of Americans without adequate access to care or burdened by insurmountable costs.

Reframing the narrative also means moving beyond polarized debates that pit innovation against equity, or capitalism against compassion. The two are not mutually exclusive. A well-designed healthcare system can leverage market principles to expand access and improve outcomes without undermining the innovation that defines American medicine. This requires recognizing that reform is not about dismantling what exists but about rethinking how it operates.

The narrative must evolve to embrace the complexity of healthcare. It is not a moral failure or an irredeemable system, but a deeply human one—shaped by competing priorities, entrenched interests, and societal values. By shifting the focus from blame to possibility, we can pave the way for a more constructive dialogue. A system designed to prioritize both excellence and equity is not beyond reach; it simply demands a new way of thinking, one that balances what works with what must change.

BALANCING THE THREE PILLARS: INNOVATION, ACCESS, AND SUSTAINABILITY

A future-oriented vision for U.S. healthcare must rest on three interconnected pillars: innovation, access, and sustainability. These elements, while often treated as competing priorities, are in fact mutually reinforcing when thoughtfully aligned. Striking this balance requires a nuanced approach that preserves the strengths of the current system while addressing its most critical flaws.

Innovation has long been the hallmark of American healthcare. From lifesaving drugs to groundbreaking medical technologies, the U.S. leads the world in advancing the frontiers of medicine. This is not an accidental outcome but the result of a system that rewards creativity and competition. However, the pursuit of innovation cannot remain unchecked by considerations of access. The development of cutting-edge treatments holds little value if they remain out of reach for the majority. True progress lies not just in the ability to cure but in ensuring that cures are available to those who need them most.

Access, therefore, must be elevated as a parallel priority. Expanding coverage, addressing healthcare deserts, and reducing cost barriers are not merely ethical imperatives; they are essential to the system's legitimacy. A healthcare system that excludes large segments of the population undermines its own potential, wasting resources on avoidable emergencies and perpetuating cycles of poor health that burden families and economies alike. Access is not an enemy of innovation but its natural complement, ensuring that the benefits of progress are shared broadly.

Sustainability is the third pillar, anchoring the other two. Without a focus on long-term cost efficiency, both innovation and access will falter under the weight of an unsustainable financial model. This requires systemic reforms to reduce administrative waste, realign incentives, and adopt preventative care strategies that mitigate chronic illnesses before they escalate. It also demands a cultural shift, encouraging both providers and patients to embrace practices that prioritize health outcomes over volume-based care.

Balancing these pillars does not mean compromising excellence for equity or stifling innovation for affordability. Instead, it calls for a reimagined framework where these priorities work in harmony. With the right incentives and policies, the U.S. can build a healthcare system that leads the world not just in what it achieves but in how it delivers those achievements to all its people.

Creating a healthcare system that embodies innovation, access, and sustainability requires a collective effort from all stakeholders. Each has a distinct role to play, and meaningful progress can only emerge through coordinated actions that acknowledge their interdependencies.

The government, as both regulator and facilitator, must craft policies that incentivize positive outcomes while curbing excesses. It has the power to establish guardrails that ensure fairness in pricing, enforce transparency, and promote equitable access without stifling the competitive forces that drive innovation. Public funding for research and healthcare programs like Medicaid and Medicare must be allocated strategically, balancing immediate needs with investments in long-term health infrastructure. Policymakers must move beyond ideological gridlock and recognize their responsibility to both constituents and the system's overall stability.

Corporations, including pharmaceutical companies, insurers, and healthcare providers, hold unparalleled influence in shaping the system. They must acknowledge their dual responsibilities: to shareholders and to society. Innovation should remain a priority, but it must be pursued with a commitment to affordability and accessibility. Businesses thrive in an environment where their contributions to public health translate into trust and sustainability. This means embracing practices that prioritize efficiency, reduce waste, and align with patient-centered outcomes rather than purely profit-driven metrics.

Healthcare professionals, the system's frontline providers, are both advocates and agents of change. Their firsthand experiences with the system's inefficiencies and inequities position them uniquely to inform and lead reform efforts. Physicians, nurses, and allied health workers must continue to push for models of care that emphasize quality over quantity and holistic approaches over fragmented services. At the same time, they must collaborate with policymakers and corporate stakeholders to ensure their voices are integral to the decision-making process.

Patients, often perceived as passive participants, are in fact the system's foundation. Their choices, behaviors, and demands influence everything from market dynamics to public policy. A well-informed and engaged patient population is critical to driving change. However, this requires education, transparency, and access to resources that empower individuals to take an active role in their health. Personal accountability must be matched with systemic support, ensuring that patients are neither blamed for their circumstances nor excluded from solutions.

Together, these stakeholders form a complex ecosystem, each with its unique responsibilities and incentives. The challenge lies in fostering collaboration without compromising the core values each group represents. A system in which all stakeholders work toward shared goals—leveraging their strengths while holding one another accountable—has the potential to achieve a balance that serves both the individual and the collective.

Charting a Course for Change

The U.S. healthcare system, as it stands, reflects the intricate web of values, priorities, and compromises that define the nation. Yet, recognizing this reality is not an endpoint but a starting point for action. The system is not immutable; it is a human construct, and as such, it can evolve. But meaningful change requires collective will, pragmatic vision, and an unwavering commitment to balance innovation, access, and sustainability.

Policymakers must transcend partisan divides to create reforms grounded in evidence rather than ideology. Incremental changes—such as capping drug prices, expanding telehealth, and incentivizing preventative care—are practical steps that can pave the way for broader transformations. At the same time, regulatory frameworks must adapt to ensure that new technologies and treatment modalities enhance equity rather than exacerbate disparities.

Corporations must shift their focus from short-term profits to long-term stability. Embracing models that reward value rather than volume, investing in community health initiatives, and committing to transparent pricing are not just ethical imperatives but strategic necessities in a world increasingly demanding accountability. By demonstrating a willingness to prioritize public good alongside shareholder returns, industry leaders can help restore trust and legitimacy to the system.

Healthcare professionals are called to lead not only at the bedside but also in the boardroom and the halls of power. Their expertise and advocacy are essential in crafting policies and practices that align with patient needs. By uniting their voices, providers can counteract the forces that prioritize profit over care and advocate for a system that respects their labor and their patients' dignity.

Patients, too, have a role to play. Civic engagement—whether through voting, advocacy, or informed decision-making—can exert pressure on policymakers and corporations to prioritize reform. By demanding transparency, accountability, and fairness, individuals can help drive the system toward greater equity and responsiveness.

The path forward requires a cultural shift as much as a structural one. It calls for a collective acknowledgment that healthcare is not merely a commodity or a privilege but a foundational element of societal well-being. To chart this course, each stakeholder must embrace their responsibility to foster a system that reflects the best of American values—innovation tempered by compassion, competition balanced with fairness, and individual success woven into collective progress.

Toward an Equitable and Innovative Future

The complexities of the U.S. healthcare system may seem insurmountable, but they also present an opportunity for reinvention. A system that has driven unparalleled advancements in medicine and technology is equally capable of evolving to meet the demands of a changing society. The future of healthcare in America does not lie in abandoning its core principles but in reimagining how those principles can serve a broader, more inclusive purpose.

As the nation grapples with questions of access, affordability, and sustainability, the potential for meaningful reform remains within reach. Each challenge presents an opportunity: technological innovations can be harnessed to close gaps in care, policy reforms can address inequities without stifling competition, and cultural shifts can foster a collective commitment to health as a shared value.

Progress will not come without struggle. Change demands perseverance, collaboration, and the courage to challenge entrenched norms. Yet history demonstrates that even the most complex systems can adapt when guided by the determination to create a better future. By embracing this possibility, stakeholders at every level—government, industry, healthcare professionals, and patients—can transform the system into one that not only reflects the nation's values but elevates them.

In the end, the U.S. healthcare system is a reflection of its people: innovative, resilient, and capable of remarkable transformation. The path forward will require hard choices and unwavering resolve, but it also offers the promise of a system that works not just for some but for all. With a shared vision and collective effort, the nation can move toward a future where healthcare is a cornerstone of both individual well-being and societal progress.

Discover more

Autor

Other books

www.ingramcontent.com/pod-product-compliance
Lightning Source LLC
Chambersburg PA
CBHW031611210526
45464CB00004B/1531